SAVING YOUR SKIN

Prevention, Early Detection, and Treatment of Melanoma and Other Skin Cancers

By Barney J. Kenet, M.D.
and Patricia Lawler

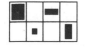

Four Walls Eight Windows, New York/London

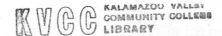

© 1994 Barney Kenet and Patricia Lawler

Published in the United States by:
Four Walls Eight Windows
39 West 14th Street, room 503
New York, N.Y., 10011

U.K. offices:
Four Walls Eight Windows/Turnaround
27 Horsell Road
London, N51 XL, England
First printing April 1994.

Nothing in this book should be construed to imply any endorsement of the treatments described in this book. Nor is this book, or any part of it, intended to replace the services of a physician. The authors and publisher make no warranty, express or implied, with respect to the material described within this book.

Library of Congress Cataloging-in-Publication Data:
Kenet, Barney, 1960-
Saving your skin: early detection, treatment, and prevention of melanoma and other skin cancers/
Barney Kenet and Patricia Lawler.
p.   cm.
Includes bibliographical references and index.
ISBN: 1-56858-009-6
1. Melanoma—Popular works. 2. Skin—Cancer—Popular works. I. Lawler, Patricia, 1959-   II. Title. RC280.M37K46   1994
616.99'477—dc20   94-3185
CIP

Text design by Quay Design Group

10 9 8 7 6 5 4 3 2

Printed in the United States

Table of Contents

Acknowledgements

Preface

Introduction

Chapter 1
The Melanoma Time Bomb 1

Chapter 2
Section **I** The Skin: A Window and a Wall 19
Section **II** The Structure and Function of Human Skin 24

Chapter 3
Melanoma and the Nature of Cancer 28

Chapter 4
Identifying Melanoma 42

Chapter 5
Screening for Melanoma 56

Chapter 6
After Identification-Biopsy 63

Chapter 7
Staging of Melanoma 68

Chapter 8
Choosing Your Doctor 80

Chapter 9
When Melanoma Spreads to the Lymph Nodes 89

Chapter 10
If Melanoma Returns 98

Chapter 11
Traditional Treatments for Advanced Melanoma 106

Chapter 12
Experimental Treatments for Advanced Melanoma 127

Chapter 13
Emotional Aspects of Melanoma 146

Chapter 14
Safe Sun Habits for a Lifetime of Healthy Skin 161

Glossary 180

Appendix 184

Index 197

Acknowledgments

We are most grateful to those who agreed to share their experience with melanoma with us. Often, their stories were very personal and sometimes painful, but their willingness allowed us to write a book that speaks, we hope, to every person affected by this disease. Sharon Pratt was especially helpful in connecting us with melanoma patients around the country. Her enthusiasm and concern, no doubt, is an inspiration to everyone who knows her. Sharon's support for this project reinforced our belief that this book was important.

Our new friend Dr. Thomas B. Fitzpatrick deserves a hand. He was one of the first people we told about the book when it was still just an idea. His response was overwhelmingly positive and encouraging. His lifelong efforts at describing melanoma, especially in its early stages, have made our task in this book possible.

Several fine doctors contributed to our understanding of melanoma and provided us with insight. Dr. Anthony Albino, Dr. Larry Nathanson, Dr. Michael Mastrangelo, Dr. Alan Houghton, Dr. Jean-Claude Bystryn, Dr. Arthur Rhodes, and Dr. Jon Levenson deserve thanks for spending their time discussing the complexities of melanoma with us. Each of them has studied and contributed to a specific aspect of this disease and its treatment. More importantly, each of them has demonstrated a generous spirit by their willingness to share their wisdom and experience. We appreciate their efforts.

Thanks to Miryam Lopez-Briones Verges, an artist with great talent, who has demonstrated some of her special skills with the graphs in this book. As usual, she was patient and understanding with our wishes. John Mahoney, another young artist, provided the skin examination illustrations.

The color photographs of melanoma were provided by Dr. Joseph Bikowski. We acknowledge his gracious cooperation and efforts on our behalf.

We were lucky to have a crackerjack researcher, Cheryl Colbert, M.D. She was able to find the sometimes obscure, but interesting background information just when we needed it most. Thanks also to Hilory Wagner.

To John Oakes for his ceaseless criticism, worry and praise. He is to be credited for coming up with the concept for this book and then allowing us the freedom to explore all the issues we felt were important.

Robert Kenet, M.D., Ph.D., a visionary scientist who cultivated our interest in melanoma, is to be thanked. He has become a world authority in the field and we owe him a debt of gratitude for his inspiration. He painstakingly reviewed this manuscript for medical accuracy. Every one of his comments made a valuable contribution.

Tom Gold, Esq., was an invaluable help. He was our layperson barometer who told us when we were making things too complicated. Thanks to him, the book will be more understandable to people without a medical education.

Thanks to John Werber, M.D., our traveling companion, for his good humor.

Finally, to Monica, Stacia, Brian, Ben and Andrew, Catherine and Justin and V. Scott Prieto we are grateful. Thanks also to Don Razzano, a staunch supporter and loyal friend.

Preface

"Fear has big eyes." This Russian proverb describes our worry about cancer—of the breast, ovary, uterus, and cervix in females; prostate in males; the lung, pancreas and colon in both sexes, and on and on.

Doctors and patients are seeking ways to prevent cancer and to find clues to the early stages of cancer because timely diagnosis often means "cure." Of course, prevention is the best medicine, but at present this approach applies only to a few cancers for which we know the primary cause: lung cancer, where smoking is the culprit, and melanoma skin cancer, which is in some way related to sunlight exposure in certain susceptible populations.

Early detection is feasible for victims of a few serious cancers through mammography for breast cancer, endoscopy for colon and rectal cancers and Pap smears for cervical cancer. These tests, however, involve the patient's willingness to undergo special testing.

Saving Your Skin, written for the layperson, describes the early detection of melanoma and melanoma precursors by using only our eyes. The features of melanoma or pre-melanoma are there before us, in full view. Self-recognition of pre-melanomas and melanomas is crucial, because melanoma skin cancer is now increasing at a rate approaching epidemic proportions.

In the 1990s, however, melanoma of the skin has an excellent survival record. This is the direct result of the capability to recognize the features of small, seemingly innocuous melanomas which have no symptoms. These features—outlined in this book—often went unnoticed or disregarded in the past by both patients and physicians. As a result of new research, there is earlier diagnosis of melanoma and now a high cure rate. More than an 88-percent five-year survival rate has been achieved through the education of physicians and other health-care professionals. *Saving Your Skin* is the first detailed and complete educational treatise on melanoma written specifically for the layperson, so that anyone can learn to recognize early melanoma of the skin.

Saving Your Skin is primarily concerned with teaching people to understand melanoma skin cancer in order to assure early detection and cure—a realistic goal because, as the well-known dermatopathologist Dr. A. Bernard Ackerman has said, "No one should die of melanoma." That is to say that melanoma, among all the serious cancers, is to a unique degree curable. It is one of the very few cancers for which a non-specialist can, with a few guidelines, easily identify the earliest stages.

Saving Your Skin could save your life or the life of a close family member, a colleague or a neighbor.

Thomas B. Fitzpatrick, M.D., Ph.D., D.Sc.(Hon.)
Wigglesworth Professor of Dermatology, Emeritus
Chairman Emeritus, Department of Dermatology
Harvard Medical School, Massachusetts General Hospital
January, 1994

INTRODUCTION

If you picked up this book, you may already know what melanoma is and want to know more. Perhaps you are intrigued by the way the sun can damage our skin and lead to cancer. You may be one of the many people at risk for skin cancer, either because of your family history, a fair complexion or excessive sun exposure. You or someone you love may have been diagnosed with melanoma. In any case, this book will provide you with answers about this increasingly common and complex disease. On a more personal level, you will read about people who have triumphed over melanoma and others who are still struggling with it.

If you are not familiar with the word "melanoma" you are probably at least aware that moles and freckles can sometimes turn cancerous. What you may not know, however, is that melanoma is the most dangerous type of skin cancer. Unlike other types such as basal cell and squamous cell carcinoma, melanoma has a potent tendency to spread and kill.

Melanoma arises from the malignant transformation of melanocytes, the cells that provide your skin with its color. When clusters of these malignant cells develop, their changing nature may be revealed on the skin's surface as a dark, irregularly-shaped mole. In other situations, a normal looking mole may begin to change. It may darken, grow larger, and spread outside its borders which may become notched or irregular. Unlike almost any other type of cancer, its warning signs are easy to see.

Melanoma is one of the simplest cancers to cure if found early, but later on, one of the most difficult.

Much of this book is devoted to helping you identify melanoma and get appropriate treatment before it begins its insidious spread. This is the area where the greatest good can be accomplished and the most lives saved. However, other aspects of this disease are explored as well. Vaccine therapy to prevent advanced disease is the subject of intense research around the world. It holds promise to become one of the most exciting breakthroughs in the treatment of melanoma. Patients undergoing vaccine and other types of experimental therapy have shared their experiences for this book. Their courage and foresight have provided the scientific community with a fund of knowledge that allows this valuable research to continue.

Like many types of cancer, the exact cause of melanoma is unknown. Ultraviolet radiation from the sun is considered to be one of the greatest factors in its development. Besides the sun, heredity, immunosuppression and other at-present-unknown causes have contributed to the rise of melanoma.

Do we really need another book about cancer? In bookstores and libraries today there are dozens of titles on breast and prostate cancer as well as comprehensive general cancer books. We wrote *Saving Your Skin* because there is no single book devoted to melanoma for the layperson. Most of the current books on skin focus primarily on cosmetic considerations—such as the latest treatment for wrinkles, age spots and varicose veins. While this area of skin health is important and interesting, it does not fill the void for information about a disease whose appearance on the skin is only the beginning.

Any doubts about the need for this book were dispelled when we began speaking to melanoma patients. Every one of them told us how they had searched for—but didn't find—an understandable explanation of this disease and its treatment. Many doctors told us that they had often wished for a straightforward but authoritative text they could give their melanoma patients. One patient told us of her frustration at going to the library after her diagnosis only to be confused by complicated medical books that gave a cold and clinical explanation of a condition that would affect her for the rest of her life.

Every day in his dermatology practice, Barney meets people who wonder about a particular mole or freckle. Is it cancerous? Should it be removed? What are the warning signs? These concerns seem warranted as we witness the increase of melanoma around the world. *Saving Your Skin* will also serve to reassure people that not every spot or mole is a melanoma. After all, peace of mind is an essential part of a person's overall health. We hope this book will contribute to that facet of a person's life as well.

We hope that the information about early detection in this book will alert many to the window of opportunity that exists to identify his or her changing mole and increase the chance for cure to almost one hundred percent.

Like all serious diseases, melanoma affects not only the patient but his or her family as well. William was a patient who was 83 when he first came to see Barney about some age spots on his balding head. He was spry, alert and accompanied by his dear friend Doris, who was 67. From the look of William's skin, it was clear that he was a sun lover, and in fact, he enjoyed rummaging around outdoor flea markets and was an avid fisherman. For the most part he looked healthy, except for a dark mole with jagged edges that didn't appear normal. That mole turned out to be malignant melanoma. Because the malignancy had not invaded deeply into his skin, his prognosis was excellent. William was pleased, but not as much as Doris was. Later, she told Barney that her first husband had died of melanoma, and she realized that William's life had been saved because his disease was caught early.

This story and those of melanoma patients in the following pages attest to both the progress we have made in fighting this disease, and also the distance we have yet to go. We are confident that through education, early detection, and treatment we can reduce the suffering and deaths this disease exacts. We hope that this book will work towards that end.

Barney J. Kenet, M.D.
and Patricia Lawler

New York, New York

December, 1993

CHAPTER 1

The Melanoma Time Bomb

Melanoma, the deadliest type of skin cancer, is on the rise. Its rate of increase is rising more rapidly than any other malignancy. Some experts predict that it may soon become the third most common form of cancer in the United States if measures to control it are not instituted.

The good news is that melanoma can be cured in its early stages. It is easy to spot and simple to remove. Expensive technology isn't needed. Not even a blood test is required. The early signs are usually visible to the naked eye. The only thing we need to know is what to look for. That information is easy to learn and remember. With it, the "melanoma time bomb" can be defused.

No one likes to talk about cancer, especially the type of cancer that affects people in the prime of their lives. No one enjoys thinking about an illness for which treatment is difficult and the cure elusive. No one wants to be reminded of the fact that the chance of being struck by the disease increases because of old habits. But these are the facts about melanoma.

Hours of sunbathing and frequent sunburns, especially in childhood, and other still unknown factors account, in part, for the increase in melanoma among fair-skinned people. Faced with the rising number of melanoma cases, the medical community has begun a full-scale effort to educate the public about sun protection (primary prevention) and early detection (secondary prevention).

Every year, thousands of lives are cut short by melanoma. Many others, apparently free of disease after surgical removal of their malignant mole, face an uncertain future. Melanoma is well known for its tendency to return in other parts of the body after years without any symptoms.

The brief stories that follow illustrate how delay and ignorance can make the difference between life and death.

> *Though fair-skinned, Tony rarely wore a T-shirt or used sunscreen during his many summers as a beach lifeguard. In his early thirties, he noticed a dark changing mole on his shoulder. Although he saw a doctor who recommended that the mole be removed, Tony never returned for follow-up care. At 37, with a wife and children, Tony began having difficulty breathing. Tests revealed a tumor in his lung that had spread from the untreated mole. He died from the disease nine months later.*

> *Charlotte, a successful attorney in her 30s, had a large number of freckles and moles on her body. She vacationed in Florida every year and invariably burned. When she couldn't get away for a vacation, she visited a tanning salon to keep her skin brown. She thought a tan looked "sexy." A mole on her back began to bleed and itch. Finally Charlotte saw a doctor, but the cancer had already spread to her lymph nodes. She has undergone two extensive surgeries and faces a high risk that the melanoma may return in another part of her body.*

Although these stories are frightening, the truth is that melanoma is a curable cancer. There are, however, no miracle drugs that can cure it in its advanced stages. Melanoma success stories depend on early detection, as this hopeful profile illustrates:

> *Elaine, six months pregnant and a busy mother of a three year old, noticed a mole on the top of her foot "that just didn't look right." It started to grow and change over a few months. Having read about the early warning signs of melanoma, Elaine presented the growing spot to her dermatologist. The mole was completely removed and tested, revealing "melanoma in situ," the very earliest form of melanoma—four years later, she is healthy and considered cured.*

The Statistics on Melanoma

Today there are 300,000 people in the United States who have had or are now afflicted with melanoma. Consider these statistics:

- Melanoma is the most frequent cancer among women aged 25 to 29, and the second most frequent (after breast cancer) among women aged 30 to 34.
- In 1993, approximately 32,000 Americans will be diagnosed with melanoma and 6,800 will die of it.
- Melanoma is now the seventh most common type of cancer in the U.S. and may become as common as colon cancer (presently the third most common malignancy) if steps are not taken to control it.
- The death rate from melanoma has tripled in the past four decades.
- Twenty-five percent of melanoma cases occur in people 39 years old or younger.
- Although the United States' population increased ten percent from 1980 to 1987, the number of melanomas increased 83 percent.

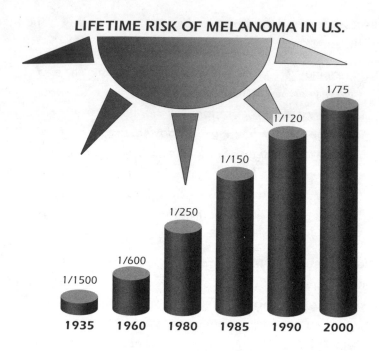

LIFETIME RISK OF MELANOMA IN U.S.

1/75 — 2000
1/120 — 1990
1/150 — 1985
1/250 — 1980
1/600 — 1960
1/1500 — 1935

Source: The Skin Cancer Foundation

Researchers at the New York University Melanoma Cooperative Group report that the lifetime risk of contracting melanoma in 1980 was one in 250; by the year 2000 the risk is predicted to climb to one in 75. Compare that with 1935, when the lifetime risk of melanoma was only one in 1,500. The N.Y.U. group further documents dramatic increases in melanoma in particular parts of the country. For example, there was a 340 percent increase in risk between 1969 and 1978 for Caucasians living in southern Arizona.

While other types of cancer—such as breast, lung, and prostate cancer—occur with greater frequency, melanoma demands close attention. It strikes and kills young to middle-aged people. On average, for each death from melanoma, more than 17 years of potential life before age 65 are lost.

The History of Melanoma

Although the rise of melanoma is a relatively new phenomenon, the disease has plagued humanity for many years. The skulls of Incan mummies some 2,400 years old show signs of the disease. One of the first official mentions of malignant moles dates to the fifth century B.C.

It was not until the 19th century, however, that important discoveries about melanoma began to emerge. Robert Carswell, a London physician, is attributed with first using the term melanoma in 1838 to describe pigmented malignant tumors, but other scientists during that time were also publishing accounts of the disease. William Norris, another Englishman, noted in 1857 that melanoma seemed to occur in "persons who have moles on various parts of their body." It has only been in more recent times that scientists have begun to understand the complex biology of this cancer. Despite progress in understanding melanoma, a cure in its advanced stages has eluded physicians.

Melanoma in Australia

The history of the colonization of Australia sets a striking scenario for the melanoma time bomb described by epidemiologists today. The explosive increase in melanoma there results mainly from the migration of fair-skinned individuals to Australia's sunny climates.

On January 26, 1788, Captain Arthur Phillip landed on the coast of Australia and founded the infant colony of New South Wales. He brought with him 717 convicts and some 300 free countrymen from his native England. Although the primary intention of the British government was the establishment of a penal colony in the sun-drenched territory, Captain Phillip encouraged his fellow countrymen to travel and settle there. By 1829, the entire continent was claimed by the British.

In the 1850s, gold was discovered in Australia and a new wave of Irish and Scottish immigrants arrived to find their fortune. The intermingling of the European pioneers helped to produce a "distinctively Australian stock" from which Asians were excluded as the result of immigration restrictions. The influx of fair-skinned foreigners from cloud-covered lands far from the equator created an unintended health problem that is reaching epidemic proportions.

Today, Queensland, Australia has the highest incidence of melanoma in the world. In the years between 1967 and 1977, the incidence of malignant melanoma in Australia doubled. In 1966, the annual incidence of melanoma was 16 per 100,000 individuals; by 1986 the incidence rate nearly tripled. The increase in melanoma in Australia has resulted in an increased death rate from the disease. Recent information suggests that mortality may be leveling off as the result of intensive efforts at educating the population about early detection and the dangers of the sun.

A recent study compared the incidence of death from melanoma between native Caucasian Australians and immigrants. Whites born in Australia had a higher incidence of melanoma than immigrants, but the earlier the age an immigrant arrived in Australia, the greater the risk of death from melanoma. The risk was especially high among immigrants from the British Isles, Austria, Germany and the Netherlands. Scientists believe that these statistics demonstrate that exposing fair-skinned people, especially children, to ultraviolet radiation from the sun increases their risk of melanoma. This study provides convincing evidence of the strange phenomenon in which sun exposure in childhood sets off what epidemiologists call the "melanoma time bomb" that explodes years later.

Confronted with these dangerous health trends, Australians have become the education leaders in the war against melanoma. Their "Slip, Slap and Slop" campaign (Slip on a T-shirt, Slap on a hat, and Slop on sunscreen) is beginning to affect attitudes about sunbathing. The desire for a suntan among Australians is on a downward trend. Advertisers of suntan lotions, recognizing the change in attitudes among Australians, now feature pale models instead of bronze ones to sell their products. These developments may signal the beginning of new health consciousness for the population "down under" and set an example for people around the world.

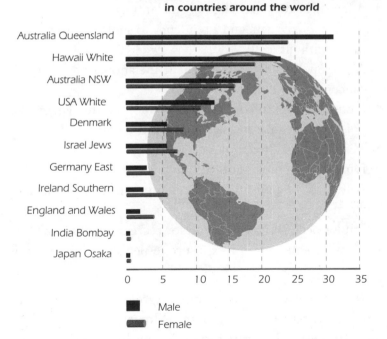

MELANOMA PER 100,000 PERSONS
in countries around the world

Source: Balch, Charles M. et al., Cutaneous Melanoma. Philadelphia: J.B. Lippincott, 1992, p. 14.

Risk Factors For Melanoma

The alarming rate at which melanoma is increasing has led to a search for its risk factors. Some of these, like hair color and genetic makeup, cannot be changed. Others factors, such as exposure to sunlight, can be modified and may help decrease your risk.

Knowing the risk factors associated with melanoma is important for two reasons. First, identifying those persons who are at a higher-than-average risk allows doctors to know which groups need to be followed and observed closely for early changes in the skin. Secondly, risk factors allow you to know what type of behavior to avoid if you want to decrease your chances of developing a melanoma.

Below are a list of risk factors for melanoma:

- A family history of malignant melanoma.
- Fair skin, light hair, and a tendency to sunburn easily and to tan with difficulty.
- A personal history of malignant melanoma or other skin cancer.
- Unusual "atypical" or "dysplastic" moles (often larger than 1/4-inch, irregular in shape and multi-colored).
- Many flat or raised moles on the body.
- Large brown moles at birth (congenital nevi).
- A history of painful or blistering sunburns, especially when young.
- Indoor occupations and outdoor recreational habits.
- Considerable outdoor exposure, especially while living in sunny regions.

Researchers are not in complete agreement about the relative importance of each factor. However, having one or more of these risk factors increases your lifetime risk.

Family History

In 1820, the English physician William Norris described a patient with melanoma whose father had died of the same disease 30 years earlier. Another case he reported involved two siblings from a set of triplets who developed melanoma at the same age on practically the same part of the body. From these anecdotal cases, Dr. Norris came to the conclusion that heredity might play a role in the development of the disease.

Accurate analysis of the inherited nature of melanoma depends on more than a few case histories, though. Towards that end, doctors at the University of Texas have studied more than 2,000 cases of melanoma to determine its tendency to run in families. The researchers concluded that there is a direct heritable pathway from parent to child. It is now estimated that approximately eight to twelve percent of all cases of malignant melanoma of the skin occur within family groups.

Personal History of Melanoma

If you had melanoma in the past, you have a five times greater-than-average risk of developing it again. The risk may even be higher in affected members of melanoma-prone families. If you have been diagnosed with any other type of skin cancer, you may be at an increased risk for melanoma as well.

Sunburns and Skin Types

Based on a number of large studies like the Australian one described above, scientists now think that melanoma in fair-skinned people is in part caused by sun exposure. It is critical to understand how vulnerable certain skin types are to ultra-violet radiation. From an early age, most people are aware how their skin reacts to sunlight. After several hours on the beach, some people turn pink, others brown, and others hardly change color at all. Many people have sun-sensitive skin. By young adulthood, half the Caucasian population has experienced at least one serious sunburn. Perhaps we don't feel the effects of a long day at the beach until evening, when our skin stings and burns, clues that we might have overdone it. In fact, the appearance of a sunburn usually begins six hours after exposure, peaks at 24 hours, and fades within 48 to 72 hours. Our skin may be burned before we actually realize it. It is equally important to understand that our sunburn fading doesn't mean that our skin has completely healed. Damage to the skin from the sun accumulates over time and adds up to an increased melanoma risk.

Dr. Rona MacKie of Scotland, a leading melanoma expert, has studied the correlation between severe sunburn and the development of melanoma. In an interview with *Dermatology Times*, she said that "a bad sunburn, whether you are a child or an adult, is not a good idea and, if repeated, is a risk factor for melanoma."

The "healthy glow" of a summer tan is a misnomer, because the sun in fact damages our skin. It is estimated that 90 percent of our skin's aged appearance is the result of sun exposure. This is known as *photoaging*. If you compare the skin on your arm to other areas of the body that aren't exposed, you can feel and see the difference.

Certain types of skin are more likely to be damaged by the sun. Dr. Thomas B. Fitzpatrick, Chairman Emeritus of the Department of Dermatology at Harvard Medical School, is a pioneer in the study of skin diseases. Today any young dermatologist eager to diagnose a perplexing case will undoubtedly refer to Dr. Fitzpatrick's *Dermatology in General Medicine*, the Bible of dermatology.

Dr. Fitzpatrick has categorized skin into six "phototypes," based on reactions to the sun. Types I and II (described below) are recognized as high-risk melanoma skin types. According to Dr. Fitzpatrick, persons with skin types I and II should never sunbathe or do outdoor work without appropriate clothing. He warns that even people with brown or black hair and dark eyes can be skin type I or II. Anyone with type I or II, regardless of hair or eye color, should use sunscreen whenever they go outdoors.

Human Skin Phototypes

Reaction to Sun	Unexposed Skin Color
I. Always burns easily, never tans	White
II. Always burns easily, tans minimally and with difficulty	White
III. Burns minimally, tans gradually and uniformly	White
IV. Burns minimally, always tans well	Light brown
V. Rarely burns, tans profusely	Brown
VI. Never burns, tans profusely	Dark brown or black

Ethnic Background

Individuals with a northern European heritage (generally those of Anglo-Saxon or Scandinavian descent) are at a higher risk for melanoma than descendants of southern Europeans. There is conflicting information about whether someone with light hair from a southern European background is at any greater risk; however, light hair in general, especially red hair, is a well-known risk factor. Usually, skin that freckles easily and burns in the sun is more susceptible to damage. This may place you at an increased risk for melanoma.

Moles and Melanoma

In eighteenth-century France, moles were a fashion statement. Ladies applied "mouches pour bal" to their faces with black plasters designed as stars, circles or crescents. Contemporary scientific insight has changed our attitudes. One researcher has commented, "We are unromantically moved by any of them. They have given us nothing but trouble."

Most moles, marks, and freckles on the skin pose no threat to a person's health. They are merely collections of pigmented cells. They can be flat or raised, pink, tan or brown. No one is certain why a mole—also called a *nevus* (plural *nevi*) appears on the skin. Infants generally have no moles on their body, but by the age of 25, most people have developed approximately 40 of them. These types of moles are called *acquired nevi*. As a person ages, his or her moles tend to flatten and disappear.

Moles are a risk factor for melanoma partly because of the chance that one may become malignant. Thus, the more moles a person has the greater the chance one may develop into a melanoma, according to one theory.

There is some controversy in the medical community over how many melanomas arise "de novo," meaning without a pre-existing mole. At present, there is no clear answer. Certain types of irregular moles are strongly associated with melanoma. These "high-risk" moles are discussed in the following section.

Atypical Moles

For many years doctors called an irregular mole a *dysplastic nevus*. Today, they are called *atypical* moles. Although there is controversy regarding its exact definition, an atypical mole is generally described as a mole that is greater than five millimeters in size (about 1/4 inch across) with irregular or fuzzy edges. Atypical moles range from tan to dark brown and may have a pink background.

An atypical mole is sometimes called a *precursor lesion*, because it may degenerate into melanoma. Investigators also consider atypical moles to be "markers" for melanoma in general because their presence may be a sign of increased melanoma risk elsewhere on the body.

Atypical moles usually appear on the areas of the body exposed to the sunlight during sunbathing, particularly the trunk. They can also be found on areas of the body not exposed to sunlight, although this is less common.

Some families can be affected by *Familial Atypical Mole and Melanoma* (FAM-M) Syndrome. It is defined as (1) an occurrence of melanoma in one or more first- or second-degree relatives; (2) a large number of moles (more than 50), some of which are atypical and variable in size; and (3) moles that have distinctive microscopic patterns.

Individuals with FAM-M Syndrome may have a lifetime risk as high as 100 percent for developing melanoma. The National Institutes of Health recommends that broad-spectrum sunscreens or protective garments be used when sun exposure is anticipated for people in this high-risk group. The FAM-M Syndrome definition is a new way of identifying persons at high risk and could potentially lead to more effective surveillance and increased survival rates.

For those people with atypical nevi, the Skin Cancer Foundation recommends the following:

1. Write down a thorough family history of unusual moles, melanomas and other cancers to discuss with your doctor.
2. Have close relatives examined for any sign of atypical nevi or melanomas.
3. Have regular complete skin exams at intervals suggested

by your doctor.

4. Supplement medical check-ups with self-examination of the skin every month.

5. Reduce sun exposure and teach your family that excessive sun exposure may stimulate formation of new moles or may cause melanomas.

6. Check with your doctor to see if he or she recommends a set of full-body photographs so that changes can be more easily spotted, especially if family members have atypical nevi or melanoma and/or have many moles.

7. Have any abnormalities in skin growth examined promptly by your doctor.

8. Check with your physician to see if an eye examination is recommended, since moles may affect the eyes.

9. Be concerned but don't worry excessively. With regular self-examination, professional examination, and common sense there is little chance that a melanoma can grow to a threatening depth before it is detected and removed.

Other High Risk Moles

Other types of moles also carry a relatively higher risk of developing into melanoma. These are called *congenital nevi.* "Congenital" means present at birth. These moles can range in size from tiny to very large. The largest types are called *bathing trunk nevi* because of their location on the body.

Lentigo maligna, another precursor to melanoma, is a flat mark, usually on the face, occasionally with raised bumps inside it. It may have striking variations in hues of brown and black and appears like a stain on the skin. It has been described as having an irregular shape, like countries on a map, with inlets and peninsulas. It usually appears on elderly people with light skin who have had a lot of sun exposure. Because lentigo maligna can turn into a type of melanoma, it should be removed if possible.

Indoor Occupation/Outdoor Recreation: Melanoma and Lifestyle

Lifestyles can influence the risk of many types of diseases, including melanoma. When one group of people is afflicted with a disease more often than another group, its behavior is studied as a possible contributing factor. With melanoma, certain behaviors and lifestyles have been associated with an increased risk of this cancer.

Melanoma tends to strike people who work indoors and play outdoors. In addition, the incidence and death from melanoma are highest among the higher social classes and professionals. These associations are probably due to the fact that wealthier people often take vacations to sunny climates after spending many months indoors. During these trips, their skin may become exposed to intense sunlight for short periods of time. Intermittent, intense exposure to sunlight is associated with melanoma.

Pregnancy and Melanoma

The relationship between melanoma and pregnancy is not clear, but has been an area of intense investigation for a number of reasons. Hormones that affect skin color circulate at increased levels during pregnancy. More than ten percent of women experience changes in their moles in the first trimester of pregnancy. About one fourth of all patients with malignant melanoma are women of childbearing age. Finally, there are some preliminary studies which suggest that pregnant women with advanced stages of melanoma have a worse prognosis than women who are not pregnant.

Doctors are trying to determine whether pregnancy is an additional risk factor for melanoma. Until the answer to this question is known, some doctors recommend that women of childbearing age who have had melanoma should not become pregnant again for two years from the date of their diagnosis. Doctors also recommend that women who have more advanced melanoma avoid both pregnancy and the use of oral contraceptives, if possible. This precaution is based on some preliminary studies that indicate there may be accelerated growth of advanced melanoma initiated by the hormones of pregnancy.

Changes Over the Years

In the late 1960s, Dr. Thomas Fitzpatrick began to define the characteristics of early melanoma, such as border irregularity and darkening. These definitions enabled physicians to diagnose moles that needed to be removed. Forty years of experience have allowed Dr. Fitzpatrick to gain a perspective that is rare in any field.

Dr. Fitzpatrick recalls that twenty years ago, before information about the early signs of melanoma was known, it was common for patients to first see him when a mole had already begun to bleed and ulcerate, ominous signs that the disease had spread and was by then incurable. In more recent years, although the number of melanomas has increased significantly, patients now tend to see Dr. Fitzpatrick and other dermatologists earlier—and with more curable melanomas. In 1940 the five-year survival rate for melanoma was 40 percent. By 1950, the number rose to 49 percent. Today, the rate has climbed to over 85 percent.

This success is due in large part to Dr. Fitzpatrick's work in educating doctors and patients about the importance of early detection. "The spectacular improvement in the overall prognosis of cutaneous melanoma in the past two decades was achieved not by using any of the standard therapies for cancer, but by the early diagnosis of primary melanomas," he says.

Sometimes, the reporting of a dramatic increase in the incidence of a disease can be attributed to improved methods of diagnosis or detection. The increase in melanoma, however, is believed to truly reflect a rise in the absolute number of cases. Faced with this growing problem, doctors are trying to teach everyone how to detect early melanoma when it is curable.

"We are at the crossroads of reducing melanoma deaths to a small fraction," Dr. Fitzpatrick says. "It is so easy, yet we will not accomplish the goal until we can reduce the number of deaths that occur from advanced melanoma that has escaped early detection."

Dr. Fitzpatrick has challenged the medical community and the general public to defuse the melanoma time bomb. He suggests that the following steps be taken to reduce deaths from this disease:

1. The general public should be made aware that melanoma of the skin is virtually epidemic among both young adults and the elderly.
2. Early malignant moles should be discovered and properly removed.
3. The high risk population should be targeted. People with skin type I or II, people with a family history of melanoma, and people with a large number of moles or atypical moles need proper education and screening.
4. Risk factors and the importance of early detection need to be publicized.
5. All health professionals, not just dermatologists, need to be informed about melanoma.

6. Free weekly screening for the high-risk population should be implemented.

What We Can Do

Worrying is not the the answer. Gaining information about melanoma's early warning signs and reducing your sun exposure are constructive responses to the concern about this deadly skin cancer.

Melanoma has captured the attention of the medical world as its incidence increases year by year. If you or a family member fit the "melanoma profile," information about this disease should command your attention as well.

CHAPTER 2

Part 1

The Skin: A Window and a Wall

While most people do not think of their skin as an organ in the same way they think of their heart or liver, it is, in fact, the largest human organ. There are 1.85 square meters (about 20 square feet) on an average male, 1.6 square meters (about 17 square feet) on an average female. The skin accounts for 16 percent of total body weight. At its thickest, it wraps our hands and feet with a protective yet highly sensitive three to six millimeter (1/10 to 1/5 of an inch) cover, while at its thinnest, it gently protects our eyes with lids that comprise a paper-thin layer of 0.5 millimeters (1/100 of an inch). Our skin defends us from external forces (heat, cold and trauma), and reveals our reactions to internal ones (blushing and pallor).

From a baby's first contact with a mother to the tactile pleasures of sexuality, skin forms a person's connection to the world. Through a language uniquely its own, the skin communicates information about each of us—how we live, who we are, and how we feel.

Our skin is a window and a wall. In its function as a window on the body, the skin makes the presence of diseases— such as a melanoma—known. As a wall, it prevents, at least for a period of time, the invasion of malignant melanoma cells into underlying blood vessels, where the cancer can begin its deadly journey to other parts of the body.

The Skin and Our Sense of Self

The farmer's furrowed brow, a teenager's acne, a 70-year-old woman's lines and wrinkles, all reveal something about their host. The appearance of skin is significant on many levels. Historically, the color of one's skin has been a determinant of social standing and identification. Skin color has profoundly, but improperly, shaped attitudes towards equality and human rights, access to opportunity and liberty. It has been suggested that, aside from gender, the color of a person's skin has the greatest impact on the fates of individuals and entire groups.

We judge others, at least in part, on their appearance. In addition, the way we inhabit and relate to our own skin reveals a great deal about how we feel about ourselves. For thousands of years, embellishment of the skin has been part of the human experience. Ancient Egyptians and fifth-century B.C. Asians applied skin oils in religious rites, and perfumes were used in the anointment of the dead. Fragrances so enthralled sixth-century B.C. Athenians that a law prohibiting their sale was passed—and subsequently ignored.

The price of vanity was often high. Some products that were used to beautify are now known to be poisonous. As early as 400 B.C., the Greeks used lead carbonate—a substance noted for its toxicity—for face powder. Poppea, wife of the Roman emperor Nero, applied this dangerous substance to whiten her face. Sixteenth-century Italian women used arsenic to give their faces a translucent appearance. In many cultures, body piercing, tattooing and ritual scarring were used to signify an individual's endurance or bravery or to mark passage into a new phase of life. Queen Elizabeth painted faint blue lines on her forehead to create the illusion of delicate skin and feathery veins.

Similar practices continue today. Now men and women

choose cosmetic surgery to enhance their appearance. Others apply countless cosmetic and medicinal preparations that promise beauty or the fountain of youth in a tube.

Skin and Our State of Mind

Phrases such as "to save your skin," "he gets under my skin," and "skinned alive" are metaphors for the function of our skin as protector and as a vulnerable wrapping of the self. These everyday phrases reflect an interest in protecting our bodies from threatening outside elements.

The perception of our bodies begins with the perception of our skin, its color, shape, texture, elasticity, and smell. In a memoir about his lifelong battle with psoriasis, author John Updike recalls the agony of appearing different from his peers. In fact, his embarrassment over this skin condition prevented him from learning how to swim until his freshman year at college. While growing up, he was treated with lotions and followed dietary restrictions in the hopes of improving his condition.

William Carlos Williams, a physician and writer who practiced among the poorest immigrants in Rutherford, New Jersey, at the turn of the century, knew that appearance was important among his patients. In a short story entitled "The Girl With the Pimply Face" he described making a house call to see a sick baby. As he entered the tenement, he was met by a young girl. He wrote: "She had one of those small, squeezed-up faces, snub nose, overhanging eyebrows . . . and a terrible complexion, pimply and coarse." While talking with the girl, Dr. Williams learned that she had stopped going to school. He recognized that her complexion was a major source of unspoken embarrassment and he prescribed a lotion. Upon returning to the house to check up on the sick infant, Dr. Williams had a quick conversation with his second young patient:

"How's your face?"

"Gettin' better."

"My God it is," I said. *And it was much better.* *"Going back to school now?"*

"Yeah, I had tuh."

In this brief interchange between doctor and patient, the significance of healthy skin as a tool for socialization and self-esteem is apparent.

The Skin as a Sign of Health

One of the first things a physician-in-training learns is that before touching a patient, he or she should simply stand back and observe. There is much to be learned about the state of a person's health from looking at the outside first. Yellow-tinged skin may indicate jaundice, suggesting that the liver may not be functioning well. Pallor, or extreme paleness, may signify anemia, while dark patches of skin under the arms and on the neck may warn of an internal malignancy. In short, our skin reflects the state of our health, and may be the physician's first clue in reaching a diagnosis.

While a complete routine physical exam or work-up for internal illness attempts to assess the well-being of the complete body, traditional medicine has tended to omit an equally thorough examination of the skin. As the incidence of melanoma increases, dermatologists know that physicians who overlook the skin miss a potentially lifesaving part of any physical exam.

One dermatologist gives an example of what can happen when the skin is routinely ignored during examination. He was asked to see a young woman shortly after the birth of her baby. Hers had been a high-risk pregnancy, and both she and her fetus had been monitored carefully throughout the months. During her obstetrical visits, however, the woman had worn knee socks, and was never asked to remove them as they didn't interfere with her exam. A melanoma on her lower leg was never observed. By the time it was spotted, the tumor had spread to other parts of her body and her prognosis was poor. This sad case illustrates the importance of viewing the skin as a vital indicator of health and illness.

Skin: Mirror to Our Emotions

In the same way our skin sends a message about the state of our health, it may also give clues about our state of mind and emotions. Who can argue that a blush isn't as much an emotional reaction as a physical one? Many skin disorders become worse during periods of stress. The United States Army, in fact, will not accept anyone with psoriasis, fearing that the stress of combat might exacerbate the condition until it became intolerable for the soldier.

We can close our mouth, shut our eyes, cover our ears, and pinch our nose, but we can't turn off our skin. It is an organ of continuous perception. We are constantly and profoundly affected by the sensations it provides. As such, the skin is our link to the external world and is the threshold for our socialization. Ashley Montagu, in a well-known treatise entitled *Touching: The Human Significance of the Skin*, observed that tactile stimulation is essential for healthy emotional and physical development. More recent studies bear this out. The skin provides humans with the sensations necessary for survival.

Psychologists have discovered a syndrome in children known as "psychosocial dwarfism" caused by a lack of touching. Provided with all other essentials, but deprived of touch, children with the syndrome demonstrated slower learning ability and growth. As recently as 1992, dermatologists and psychologists have reported that one of the causes of infantile eczema may be lack of tactile stimulation. While lotions and medication may provide relief for this condition, the problem might have been lessened with the simple, but essential, loving acts of touching and stroking the skin.

Part 2

The Structure and Function of Human Skin

Human skin is well-designed to serve many functions. It is the farthest outpost of the immune system. It acts as a barrier against toxins, chemicals, and pollutants. Its dry outer layer inhibits bacteria from growing and reproducing on its surface, and also aids in resistance to electrical shocks.

The skin regulates heat loss and works with other organs to maintain a constant body temperature. It is also of unique importance in the production, storage, and release of Vitamin D, which is essential for the absorption of calcium and phosphorous.

The Anatomy of Skin

The skin is composed of two layers: the *epidermis*, and beneath it, the *dermis*.

The Epidermis

The epidermis is the outer layer of the skin.

The top layer of the epidermis, the *stratum corneum*, is comprised of overlapping cells that create a network of protection from the environment. The epidermis is replaced every 28 days as older cells are shed from the surface and newer cells move up from the lower level, called the *basal cell layer*.

As basal cells divide and move upwards from the basal cell layer towards the surface of the skin, they become progressively flatter and harder. Eventually, they become part of the stratum corneum as the dead cells in this outermost layer are shed. These changes are imperceptible, but evidence of this process can be found in the ring in your bathtub, which is partially made up of dead skin cells.

Also within the epidermis are *Langerhans cells*. These cells play an important immunological role in providing protection against tumors, viruses and other infections by trapping parts of these invaders and facilitating their destruction. Ultraviolet radiation damages Langerhans cells, which has led some scientists to believe that skin cancer is not caused simply by a change in cells in the epidermis, but also by a breakdown in the immune system.

The Dermis

Beneath the epidermis is the second layer of the skin, called the *dermis*. This layer contains blood vessels, lymph vessels and nerves. The dermis has two levels, an upper level called the *papillary dermis* and a lower level called the *reticular dermis*.

The greatest portion of the dermis is made up of *collagen*, which are bundles of protein that are loosely arranged in wavy bands. Collagen is also found in bones, cartilage, and tendons. Collagen and the layer of fat below it do much to cushion internal organs and bones from traumatic injuries.

Collagen provides support for the skin. As a person ages, there is a gradual decrease in the amount of collagen, which accounts in part for the appearance of wrinkles and sagging skin. For unknown reasons, women suffer a greater loss of collagen than do men. In recent years, collagen has been added to cosmetics and face creams in an effort to repair aging skin. Because the stratum corneum protects against penetration by most agents into the skin, collagen applied directly to it will do little to correct wrinkles.

Elastin is also found in the dermis. As its name suggests, elastin gives the skin its elastic qualities. The fibers that make up elastin can be stretched 100 percent or more and still return to their original size. Like a rubber band, elastin has the ability to recover without a trace of damage. Elastin is found in other parts of the body as well, such as the lungs, aorta, and Achilles tendons.

The Melanocyte: The Cell from which Melanoma Develops

The *melanocyte* is the most important skin structure for a discussion of melanoma. The malignant transformation and division of the melanocyte leads to melanoma. Located within the epidermis, the melanocyte, is a cell which produces and distributes *melanin,* the substance that gives skin and hair its color. Every person, regardless of skin color, has the same number of melanocytes. It is the amount of melanin produced by the melanoctyes which gives each person his or her unique complexion.

Melanin protects the skin from damage caused by ultraviolet radiation from the sun. Blacks are at a very low risk for skin cancer because an increased amount of melanin provides them with natural protection against ultraviolet radiation. Although a tan can protect the skin from some kinds of sun damage, the skin is injured in the process. Repeated sun exposure greatly increases the likelihood of skin cancer for fair-skinned persons.

The process that turns a healthy melanocyte into melanoma is not well understood. Most likely, this transformation is the result of more than one factor. Certainly, ultraviolet radiation from the sun is suspected to play a pivotal role. Ultraviolet light damages DNA, causes immunosuppression and may activate chemicals in the body that stimulate the chain of events leading to cancer.

In addition to giving us a defining and aesthetic cloak, our skin provides us with a protective one as well. The skin's most powerful enemy is the sun, which damages not only its appearance, but corrupts its functions.

CROSS-SECTION OF HUMAN SKIN

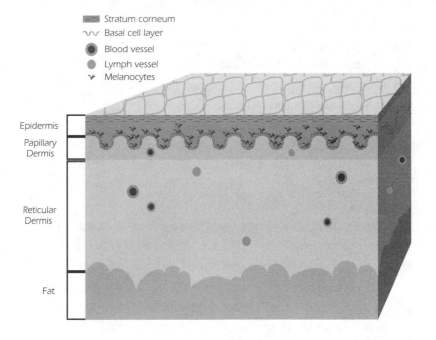

CHAPTER 3

Melanoma and the Nature of Cancer

Sixty years ago, Charles H. Mayo, a surgeon and co-founder of the famous Mayo Clinic in Rochester, Minnesota, wrote: "While there are several chronic diseases more destructive to life than cancer, none is more feared." Today, with cancer as the second leading cause of death in the United States (heart disease is first), his observation still reflects our attitudes towards the disease. Even though survival rates for many types of cancer have improved, our tendency is to view them all as incurable. One author notes that cancerphobia is deeply rooted in American culture and evokes fears which "transcend its deadliness."

Other cultures share the American fear of cancer. An Australian study determined that people who did not see a doctor until their melanomas were large and advanced had waited not because they were unaware of the disease, but because they were afraid. An understanding of the nature of cancer in general and melanoma in particular is the first step in moving beyond that fear.

"Cancer patients are terrified because they think the disease is a death sentence," says Dr. Anthony Albino, head of the Laboratory of Cell Transformation at Memorial Sloan-Kettering Cancer Center in New York. "They notice all kinds of changes, yet don't do anything about them. We need to explain to them that cancer is not the fatal disease it was thirty or forty years ago."

The facts about cancer can be difficult to understand. It is easy to "tune out" when we hear the word "cancer" mentioned. However, by learning some of the basics—about our bodies and the nature of cancer—we can begin to take control. Knowledge and control are not guarantees of success, but they are the weapons we need for a fighting chance.

The Common Characteristics of All Cancers

Cancers share similar characteristics regardless of where they strike. First, many cancers originate from a single cell which multiplies into a large number of malignant cells, commonly called a malignant tumor. This is true of melanoma. Another common trait of cancer cells is their unregulated growth. While normal cells generally grow and divide according to a programmed biological timetable, cancer cells grow in an uncontrolled manner. Not only is the growth unregulated, but given enough time, it will become invasive. This means that cancer cells tend to erode healthy surrounding tissue and burrow through it.

In some cases, malignant cells will invade adjacent tissue, blood vessels and lymphatic channels. When this occurs, the malignancy can disseminate, or spread to distant sites of the body. This is known as *metastasis*.

Since benign or non-malignant tumors never metastasize, the ability of a tumor to metastasize marks it as malignant. Metastatic cancer is more difficult to treat than a localized solitary tumor, which can often be successfully removed by surgery or eradicated with radiation.

"Having cancer is not the problem. The big problem is when it has progressed," says Dr. Albino. "Most people die of metastases, not from a primary tumor. The answer therefore is in early diagnosis."

Another common feature of cancer is *anaplasia*, which can be explained as a loss of the orderly development of cells.

The cancer cells' microscopic appearance has been described as bizarre, and haphazard. As the cancer progresses, the cells look more and more abnormal.

Cancer cells also tend to deprive normal cells of the nourishment and space they need to survive. While malignant cells multiply, more and more normal tissue is destroyed. The malignant growth has been described in one medical textbook this way: "The abnormal mass is purposeless, preys on its host and is virtually autonomous."

All the features of cancer described here are present in melanoma. Fortunately, many of the early malignant changes that take place in melanoma are in plain view, unlike other kinds of cancer in which changes take place inside the body and cannot be seen with the naked eye. It is essential, therefore, to be aware of how these changes manifest themselves on our skin, and to respond to them quickly. The more we know, and the earlier we act, the greater are our chances of a total cure.

The Causes of Cancer

Having some idea of what cancer is, the next question becomes, "What causes cancer?"

Carcinogenesis, or the development of cancer, is thought to be a multi-step process. The events that culminate in the development of cancer begin with specific changes in the DNA (deoxyribonucleic acid) of a single cell. DNA, housed within the nucleus of the human cell, contains the genetic material that makes each of us unique: our genes. Human cells contain approximately 100,000 genes, the biological unit of heredity.

Several hundred of these genes control cellular functions. When they are mutated by environmental or other factors they may turn into *oncogenes*—genes that actively promote tumor growth. In many cases, the genes that are damaged are repaired. If the change persists, however, the altered cell will divide and produce new cells that also contain altered DNA. In this setting, cancer can develop.

Tumor suppressor genes are considered to be equally if not more important than oncogenes in the development of cancer. These genes, as their name suggests, suppress the development of tumors. They are "damage control specialists" and form a complex system of responses to abnormal DNA that might otherwise lead to cancer. When these tumor suppressor genes are damaged or missing, the process which leads to cancer is more likely to occur.

Environmental factors such as chemicals or radiation can damage DNA and predispose an individual to the development of a malignancy. In addition to these factors, inherent genetic defects can increase the chance of cancer developing. These defects occur when an individual inherits a defective gene from a parent. Genetic predisposition may make a cell more susceptible to environmental agents that can cause cancer.

In summary, cancer can result from an interaction between an individual's genetic makeup and the environment in which he or she lives.

New Developments in the Field

Dr. Albino is beginning to unlock some of the mysteries regarding the genetic makeup of melanoma. He theorizes that a number of genetic and non-genetic factors result in "oncogenic transformation," meaning the changes from normal to malignant melanoma cells. His research is focusing on an array of genes that may play a role in the genesis of melanoma.

Other researchers are also trying to locate which genes are involved in the development of melanoma. Several teams of scientists are focusing on a region on chromosome 9 that is presumed to contain tumor suppressor genes associated with other types of cancer. At the University of Utah Medical Center, researchers discovered that an abnormal gene on this chromosome may determine a person's predisposition to familial melanoma. People carrying this genetic abnormality may have a fifty percent increased risk of developing the disease. This study was based on following eleven large extended families with melanoma. According to reports published by Dr. Mark H. Skolnick of the University of Utah, the discovery marks only the second time that scientists have pinpointed an inherited susceptibility to a common form of cancer. These discoveries may someday allow for early identification of people at risk of developing melanoma and also provide the foundation for new and innovative therapies.

Carcinogens

Carcinogens cause cancer. There are three main categories: chemicals, viruses, and radiation.

Proving or disproving that a substance causes cancer can take many years. In many cases, scientists rely upon epidemiological studies. Epidemiology searches for relationships between lifestyles and the incidence of a disease. This is in contrast to controlled laboratory studies in which animals are exposed to suspected cancer-causing agents to determine if cancer will develop.

Chemicals

In 1775, Sir Percival Pott discovered an increased amount of scrotal cancer among chimney sweeps. Sir Percival theorized that daily exposure to soot contributed to the higher-than-average cancer risk for these men. As a result of the findings, the chimney sweeps were ordered to bathe every day after work. This simple measure proved successful and the rate of cancer in this group declined.

Since that time, hundreds of other chemicals have been found to cause cancer. Industrial workers, because of their daily exposure, often provide the first clues that a substance may be carcinogenic. Asbestos, arsenic, coal by-products, and mustard gas have been associated with lung cancer, leukemia, and other types of cancer.

Naturally-occurring chemicals can be carcinogenic. Aflatoxin is produced by some strains of a fungus that thrives on improperly stored grains and peanuts. There is a strong correlation between aflatoxin in the diet and liver cancer. Infection with the hepatitis B virus is strongly associated with liver cancer as well, causing some scientists to hypothesize that aflatoxin and the virus collaborate in causing this cancer.

Viruses

A virus is the smallest form of living organism. It survives only by infecting other cells and using the machinery of that cell to make copies of itself. In its role as a carcinogen, a virus infects the cell and takes with it viral genes and viral enzymes. With these enzymes, the virus highjacks human DNA within the human cell and forces it to produce the building blocks of new viruses. The virally-infected cell now contains oncogenes which can ultimately lead to the formation of cancer.

Besides liver cancer, Burkitt's lymphoma (a type of lymph node cancer), cervical cancer and leukemia may be related to viruses. Strains of viruses have actually been found within the cells of these tumors.

What Causes Melanoma

Chemicals and viruses probably only play a limited role in the development of melanoma. At present, there is no evidence to suggest that dietary factors such as alcohol, coffee, and tea consumption cause melanoma. Similarly, preliminary studies examining the relationship between a high-fat diet and melanoma have had inconsistent results, but research continues in this area.

A lack of evidence, however, does *not* mean that these factors play absolutely no role in the development of melanoma, only that there is no scientific proof of it to date.

A rise in the incidence of melanoma has prompted a search for its causes. Many studies look for clues on the cellular level, while others obtain data by observing particularly melanoma-prone populations. As more information comes to light, old theories are discarded and new ones adopted.

A textbook on the causes of cancer, published in 1940, stated that "Uncleanliness, leading to stoppage of gland ducts and aided by infection and chemical irritation, is an important cause of many skin cancers. The remedy is soap and water, and scrubbing."

It went on to say, "Exposure to sunshine, winds, and irritating dust gives rise to innumerable keratoses, freckles, lentigines, pigmented warts, etc., which slowly lead to the large group of skin cancers."

Few scientists today would dream of laying the blame for skin cancer on dirt, but most would give their research forebears credit for recognizing that in some way the sun might be a culprit. Even non-scientist Ernest Hemingway knew there was some relationship between the sun and skin cancer. In the *Old Man and the Sea*, he wrote:

> *The old man was thin and gaunt, with deep wrinkles in the back of his neck. The brown blotches of the benevolent skin cancer the sun brings from its reflection on the tropic sea were on his cheek.*

Today insight into the damaging effects of the sun has allowed us to recognize that ultraviolet light may play a central role in the development of melanoma.

Ultraviolet Radiation

There are three types of radiation from the sun: ultraviolet (UV), visible, and infrared. Visible radiation provides light and allows us to see. Infrared and visible rays penetrate the skin and make us feel warm.

Ultraviolet radiation is divided into three wave bands: UVA, UVB, and UVC. Only UVA and UVB reach the earth's surface. When these two types of radiation reach our skin, they damage it. About ten percent of UVA and UVB is blocked by the top layer of our skin. The rest penetrates into its deeper layers. UVB activates melanocytes resulting in the production of melanin which produces a suntan. In people with lightcolored skin, UVB causes sunburns because there is not enough melanin to protect the skin adequately. In contrast, the effects of UVA are not readily apparent, but they show up years later in the form of wrinkles and a loss of elasticity in the skin.

Ultraviolet radiation is a complete carcinogen, which means it both initiates the malignant process and promotes its growth.

THE SUN'S RADIATION AND ITS EFFECT ON HUMAN SKIN

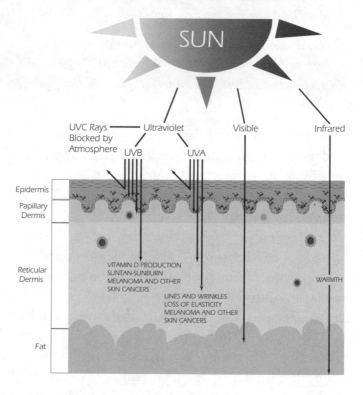

While there is little doubt that ultraviolet radiation can cause some types of melanoma, no one is sure exactly how it occurs. The most persuasive proof regarding this relationship is generally found by studying the sun exposure habits of large groups of people. For example, the 300% increase in melanoma in Scotland since 1970 is generally attributed to the increase in leisure activities among the Scots, who now spend more time on the beach during vacations. Orthodox Jews in Israel, who wear dark heavy clothing and head coverings year-round, have a significantly lower incidence of melanoma compared to non-Orthodox Israelis, who do not wear such extensive protection.

One theory attempting to explain how UV radiation may cause melanoma focuses on the observation that ultraviolet radiation induces the rapid proliferation of melanocytes, which normally divide at a slow rate when not exposed to sunlight. When melanocytes are frequently and rapidly activated because of UV exposure, a series of biochemical reactions occurs. These reactions may ultimately lead to the production of biological chemicals called growth factors—chemicals which regulate the growth of cells. The presence of these chemicals may set the stage for a pre-cancerous change.

Finally, exposure to UV radiation, particularly UVB, can weaken the immune system. Its suppression may limit the body's ability to recognize and eliminate defective cells.

The Sun and Melanoma

According to Dr. Albino, sunlight may be "all you need" to get a melanoma. The scientific community is generally in accord with the notion that sunlight harms the skin. Outside of a small genetic factor in certain families, sunlight is considered to be the primary cause of melanoma development.

Many experts agree that in the war against melanoma, the sun is our worst enemy. Avoiding exposure to the sun's rays is our best defense, and wearing sunblock and protective clothing whenever you are in the sun is the second most effective weapon.

Some Puzzling Aspects of Melanoma and the Sun

Despite the evidence linking sun exposure and melanoma, there are some troubling characteristics of the disease that have caused experts to question the relationship. First, a primary melanoma can appear on parts of the body that are rarely exposed to sunlight, such as the genitals or the soles of the feet. Dr. Arthur Rhodes, Professor of Dermatology at the University of Pittsburgh School of Medicine, suggests that the association between the sun and melanoma may not be as direct as it appears. He believes that it is important to recognize that melanoma can occur on non-sun-exposed parts of the body. To illustrate this point, he recalls an incident that occurred at the University of Pittsburgh. A second year medical resident at the hospital noticed an unusual mole in his armpit.

"He had the mole there for a long time, and both he and his wife knew there was some sort of change in the mole. They knew from the lay press that ultraviolet radiation causes melanoma. Since the mole appeared on a part of his body that didn't see the light of day, he assumed it couldn't be melanoma. It is possible that for this reason they waited too long before seeking consultation," says Dr. Rhodes. Unfortunately, the mole was malignant, the cancer spread and eventually caused the young man's death.

Dr. Rhodes points out that there is not a proportional relationship between the amount of ultraviolet exposure and the risk of malignant melanoma. Instead, it is intermittent and intense blasts of sun exposure that are associated with an increased risk.

Dr. Rhodes also believes that having many large or irregular moles is a much more significant risk factor than exposure to sunlight. "The mole factor may be impacted by ultraviolet radiation, but the mole factor, in and of itself, appears to be most significant," he says. "Having five moles, each one five millimeters [about 1/4 of an inch] or larger, is associated with a ten-fold risk, and having a dozen is associated with a forty-fold risk. Moreover, you only need one abnormal mole to have a melanoma. That mole may be in a sun-exposed part of the body, but it can also be in a protected site," he adds.

It is also important to remember that melanoma is a heterogeneous disease; there are several types that grow, look and behave differently. Certain types are closely associated with ultraviolet radiation, but in others the relationship is less clear. Dr. Rhodes thus thinks it is imprudent to generalize that all types of melanoma are caused by ultraviolet radiation. For example, the type of melanoma found most commonly among Blacks does not seem to arise from sun exposure. On the other hand, a condition called lentigo maligna, known to be caused by sun exposure, develops into invasive melanoma in about five percent of the cases. In this setting the cause and effect is fairly clear. "It is likely that some melanomas, including those associated with lentigo maligna, are initiated and/or promoted by ultraviolet radiation," says Dr. Rhodes.

As scientists struggle with the melanoma puzzle, they may discover that melanoma can develop for different reasons. Some may be due to sun exposure, while others are related to a genetic predisposition, suppression of the immune system, or a combination of all of these and even other unknown factors.

The Development of Melanoma

People who study how melanoma develops describe the process as follows. Normal skin contains healthy melanocytes. When damaged by sun exposure or some other agent, these melanocytes mutate and proliferate. As a result, a growth may appear on the skin. This growth may be less than cancerous but not entirely normal. From this growth, melanoma may develop. In other circumstances, a normal mole may degenerate into a melanoma. In its early stages, the melanoma is confined to the epidermis, the top layer of skin. At this point it can be compared to a black widow spider sitting on your skin—that hasn't bitten.

Although it is frightening to look at, it hasn't done any harm yet. To keep it from harming you, it must be removed.

Eventually some types of melanoma may begin to grow horizontally (outward from the center). The horizontal growth phase may continue for varying amounts of time depending on the type of melanoma that develops. During this phase, the melanoma can usually be removed surgically with a high chance of cure. However, if the melanoma is not removed, it has the potential to grow vertically, meaning down into the skin. This is when metastasis can occur, ultimately leading to death in many cases. The steps leading to melanoma are not inevitable. For a number of reasons, the mole may progress, remain unchanged or even regress.

The diagram below illustrates one theory about how melanoma develops. The line between horizontal and vertical growth separates curable from potentially incurable disease.

THE DEVELOPMENT OF MELANOMA

Melanocyte - The normal pigment cell
Benign mole
Atypical mole
Atypical mole cells proliferate
Melanoma in situ (early melanoma)
- -
Invasive Melanoma
Metastatic melanoma

Adapted from: Leong, S., Malignant Melamona: Advances in Treatment. Austin: R.G. Landes, 1992, p.2.

Ionizing Radiation

Another type of radiation is ionizing radiation, produced by X-rays, atomic blasts, and certain types of metals. Every part of the human body can be affected by ionizing radiation. Radiation can kill cells, blocking their ability to divide or induce mutations within them. Exposing large areas of the body to even very low doses of radiation can be quite harmful. People regularly exposed to ionizing radiation, such as miners of radioactive ores and early radiologists, were found to have higher-than-average rates of cancer.

Although there have been some studies to suggest that a relationship between ionizing radiation and melanoma exists, the results have been inconsistent and far from persuasive. As such, ionizing radiation is not considered to be a major cause of melanoma. The real environmental culprit in melanoma remains ultraviolet (UV) radiation.

CHAPTER 4

Identifying Melanoma

What Melanoma Looks Like

Many people envision cancer as a mysterious, silently growing menace inside their bodies. In too many instances, its presence only becomes apparent with the symptoms of advanced disease. With melanoma, many of the earliest signs occur right where we can see them—on the surface of our skin. If we know what to look for and how to find it, early detection and cure are possible. Each person can become his or her own "body expert" by becoming familiar with the freckles, marks and moles that form his or her personal skin landscape. If melanoma is found and removed in its earliest stage, commonly known as *melanoma in situ*, the chance for cure is almost 100 percent. If not discovered in an early stage, the chance for survival declines dramatically.

The ABCD's of Melanoma

In the vast majority of cases, a melanoma has certain features that distinguish it from normal moles. An easy-to-remember alphabetical summary of these features provides a simple but effective guide for early detection. Look for moles that have the following characteristics—they may be the first signs of melanoma:

> **A**symmetry: One side of the mole is a different shape than the other side. If you were to fold the mole in half, the borders of the two sides would not match up.

Border Irregularity: The edges of a melanoma generally appear jagged or notched.

Color Variegation: Malignant melanoma tends to have various shades of black, brown, and sometimes even pink, white, or blue in different areas. Normal moles are usually uniformly one color, from tan to dark brown.

Diameter greater than six millimeters (about 1/4 of an inch): A mole greater than six millimeters, approximately the size of a pencil eraser, should be checked, especially if it recently appeared or has changed.

Most recently, experts have added "E" for "Enlargement" to the ABCD rule. A mole growing in size carries a greater risk of being malignant than one that is not. Not every malignant mole will have every one of the ABCD's, but if you notice a mole which exhibits any one of these characteristics, you should have it promptly examined by a dermatologist.

Changes To Look For

A changing mole, whether raised or flat, may be a sign of trouble. It is therefore important to be familiar with your moles. This will allow you to recognize any differences in their appearance.

Look for the following changes:

- **Change in size,** particularly sudden or continuous enlargement.
- **Change in shape,** especially development of irregular margins.
- **Change in color,** especially a mole that becomes darker or develops a dark spot within its border or at its edge. Also look for multiple shades of dark brown, or black, red,

white, and blue; spread of color from the edge of the mole into surrounding skin.

- **Change in elevation,** for example sudden or progressive elevation of a flat freckle.
- **Change in surface,** especially scaliness, oozing, crusting, ulceration and/or bleeding.
- **Change in surrounding skin,** such as redness, swelling, or satellite pigmentation (meaning spots of color around the mole).
- **Change in sensation,** including itching, tenderness, or pain.
- **Change in consistency,** especially softening, hardening or friability (meaning the mole crumbles easily).

Normal Changes

Not every change in a mole should be a cause for alarm. Pregnancy as well as growth spurts during infancy and childhood may also cause moles to enlarge or darken. And moles can look different after they have been irritated or injured. However, these types of changes usually last no longer than two weeks after the cause has been eliminated.

The only certain way to identify a melanoma is to have the mole removed and examined under a microscope. A dermatologist has sufficient training to distinguish between moles that should be removed and others that do not need to be.

Where Melanoma is Likely to Appear

Melanoma can appear anywhere on the body, but is most frequently found on the lower legs and backs of white women and the torsos of white men, especially the back. Although no one is able to explain these patterns with absolute certainty, some experts believe that scantier clothing during sunbathing and increased recreational exposure

Asymmetry

Benign moles tend to be symmetrical, meaning an imaginary line through the center would create halves of equal shape. (figure 1)

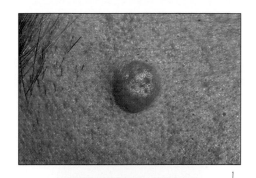

1

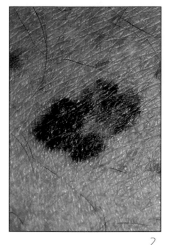

2

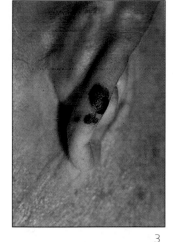

3

These superficial spreading melanomas (figures 2, 3 and 4) are asymmetrical, meaning that one half does not match the other half.

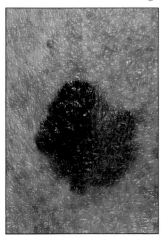

4

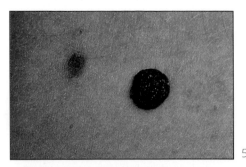

BORDER IRREGULARITY

Benign moles usually have smooth borders.

5

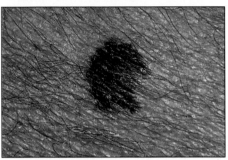

The borders of melanomas tend to be uneven or notched. Figures 6 and 7 show the notched and jagged borders of two superficial spreading melanomas.

6

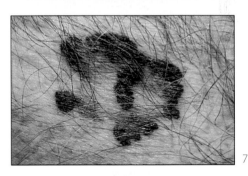

7

Figure 8 shows the irregular borders of a nodular melanoma. Note, however, that some nodular melanomas can have smooth borders. Their most distinctive characteristic is rapid growth.

8

Color VARIEGATION

A single shade of tan or brown is typical of a benign mole.

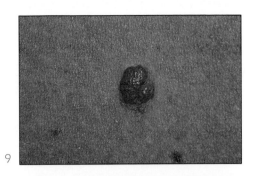

9

A melanoma usually has various shades of brown or black within it. It may also have areas of red, white or blue. Figures 10 and 11 show variations of color such as black, brown, tan, white and red.

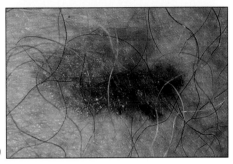

10

11

A melanoma usually has various shades of brown or black within it. It may also have areas of red, white or blue. Figures 10 and 11 show variations of color such as black, brown, tan, white and red.

Figure 12 is an example of a lentigo maligna melanoma with various shades of tan, brown and black within it.

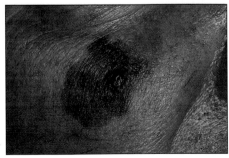

12

Diameter

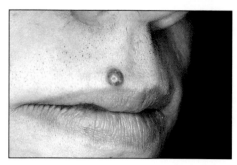

13

Benign moles are frequently less than 6 mm. (1/4 inch), about the size of a pencil eraser.

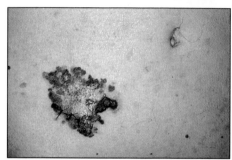

14

Melanomas, such as this large superficial spreading melanoma, are often greater than 6 mm. in size.

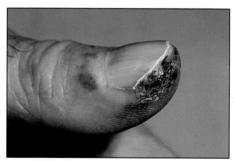

15

This acral-lentiginous melanoma involves a large portion of the thumb.

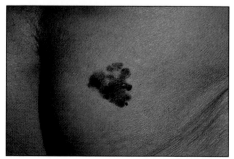

16

This advanced superficial spreading melanoma on the buttocks is almost 50 mm. across (about 2 inches).

Photographs courtesy of Joseph Bikowski, M.D.
Figure 13 photographed and provided by John Werber, M.D.

to sunlight may be contributing factors. Among Blacks and Asians, melanoma appears on the palm or sole and under the nails. In both of these ethnic groups, however, the incidence of melanoma is very low.

Most Common Locations for Melanoma on Men and Women

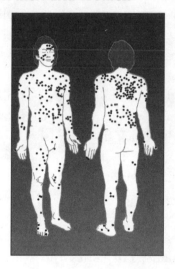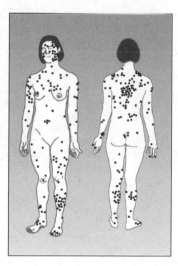

Adapted from: Fitzpatrick, Thomas B. etal., Dermatology in General Medicine. *New York: McGraw Hill, 1993, p.1080.*

Types of Melanoma

There are four sub-types of melanoma.

Superficial spreading melanoma accounts for 70 percent of all melanoma in white persons. It can be found on any part of the body, but has a tendency to appear on the legs of women and the backs of men. This type of melanoma can arise from atypical moles or other "precursor lesions" that are already on the skin. The change from an atypical nevus to a superficial spreading melanoma may sometimes take one to five years. Superficial spreading melanoma usually has an irregular border and variations in color, ranging from dark brown to black, and may have areas of blue, gray, white or pink. It is usually flat-to-slightly-raised and may be as small as six millimeters (about 1/4 of an inch).

Nodular melanoma accounts for 15 to 30 percent of melanoma. It appears most frequently on the trunk, head, and neck, and is more common in men than in women. Nodular melanoma is raised and dome-shaped and has been described as having a "cauliflower appearance." It is typically dark-brown to black and can resemble a blood blister. The edges of a nodular melanoma can be regular. Its hallmark is its rapid growth.

Lentigo maligna melanoma is less common, and is usually seen in older people, particularly women. It appears as a large irregularly-shaped brown to black flat stain (shoe polish stain) with varying colors within its border. The most common sites of lentigo maligna melanoma are areas of the body that have been exposed to the sun, such as the cheeks or nose.

Acral-lentiginous melanoma is the most common type of melanoma among Blacks, Asians, Hispanics and Native Americans. In these ethnic groups, the foot, particularly the sole or toenail, is a typical site. Other common areas are the palms and tips of the fingers. This type of melanoma usually appears as a brown-to-black flat stain with an irregular convoluted border. Under the nail, it appears as a dark stripe. Any brown to black discoloration of the cuticle and surrounding skin may also be a sign of this type of melanoma. The average age of onset is 60. Sun exposure does not seem to have any relationship to acral-lentiginous melanoma.

Other Types of Melanoma
Other types of melanoma are less common.

Mucosal melanoma appears on the mucous membranes, for

example inside the mouth, in the lining of the respiratory tract or the anal-genital region.

Amelanotic melanoma is a rare form of melanoma that is difficult to recognize. Amelanotic means without melanin or color. It appears as a pink to red growth on the skin.

Ocular melanoma begins in the eye. It accounts for three to four percent of all melanomas diagnosed. The cause of ocular melanoma is not well understood, but sunlight, viruses and chemicals may play a part in its development. Some of the signs of ocular melanoma include pigmented spots on the iris, distortion of the pupil and the presence of new blood vessels in the eye. When treated early, with surgery or radiation, ocular melanoma may be curable. Doctors are also investigating several new treatments for this condition.

Occasionally, a primary melanoma is never found although there are signs of its spread throughout the body. This is called melanoma from an unknown primary. Some doctors believe that the original melanoma may have disappeared or been destroyed, or that it began on a non-visible site such as an internal organ.

Other Types of Skin Cancer

Melanoma accounts for only a small fraction of all skin cancers, but is studied extensively because it is the deadliest. There are two other skin cancers which are much less dangerous because they tend not to spread to other parts of the body. If you have been diagnosed with either type, it is likely that you have exposed your skin to damaging ultraviolet rays. You should begin to be zealous about protecting your skin from future assaults by the sun and about examining your skin for any of the warning signs described in this chapter.

Basal cell carcinoma accounts for 60 to 70 percent of all skin cancers, with 500,000 new cases expected to be diagnosed in the United States this year. This type of skin cancer may appear as a pearl-colored, semi-translucent bump with a depressed center and rolled border. In other cases, basal cell carcinoma looks like a sore that does not heal. The face, especially the nose, forehead and ears, are common sites for basal cell carcinoma.

These growths can sometimes crust over and fall off, but that does not mean the problem has been solved. If left untreated, basal cell carcinoma can grow and destroy the surface of the skin, leaving it ulcerated and sore. In advanced cases, it can burrow under the skin, causing damage to cartilage and bone. Basal cell tumors differ from melanoma in one critical way: they rarely spread to other parts of the body (metastasize) and hence are not regarded as deadly cancers. But basal cell carcinoma should in any case be treated by a dermatologist to ensure that the tumor is properly removed.

Exposure to sunlight is the major cause of basal cell carcinoma. Less common causes are chemicals such as arsenic, or exposure to X-rays. Basal cell carcinoma is usually removed surgically, but in some cases, especially in the treatment of elderly people, radiation therapy is used. Another type of treatment is cryosurgery (freezing the tumor with liquid nitrogen). Anyone who has a history of basal cell carcinoma should use a sunscreen every day, particularly on the face and ears.

Squamous cell carcinoma is the second most common type of skin cancer, with 100,000 new cases annually. This skin cancer is most commonly found on the face, neck, bald spots, ears, and lower lip. Squamous cell carcinoma often appears on areas where there is evidence of previous sun damage, and is the skin cancer most closely associated with exposure to ultraviolet radiation. A squamous cell tumor can look like a shallow, dull-red ulcer with a raised, hardened border, or a scaly red patch with irregular borders that sometimes crusts or bleeds. These growths will often bleed when bumped.

There is a small risk that a squamous cell carcinoma will spread to distant sites of the body. This is especially true if the tumor is not treated promptly.

Besides sun exposure, squamous cell cancers can also arise from burns and chronic skin ulcers. Tumors arising from burns or ulcers are more likely to metastasize than those caused by sun damage. Although black-skinned people are less likely to develop any type of skin cancer, two-thirds of all skin cancers among Blacks are squamous cell carcinomas. Surgery is usually the best way to treat squamous cell carcinoma. It can also be treated with radiation therapy.

Common Skin Lesions

It is important to remember that not every mark on your body is dangerous. A *skin lesion* is a medical term that refers to any change or growth on the skin, such as a pimple or a wart. A mole or freckle on your skin that contains melanin is called a *pigmented lesion*. It usually poses no health threat; however, it is important to tell the difference between a normal pigmented lesion and a potentially malignant one.

The list below summarizes the more common types of normal skin lesions.

Compound Nevus: This common mole can usually be distinguished from melanoma because it is uniform in color and has well-marked, smooth borders. A compound nevus can be dome-shaped, but will still have a very regular border. Its color ranges from pink to very dark brown.

Lentigo ("liver spot"): A lentigo is a flat brown mark with a sharp border. It arises from long-term sun exposure and as such is most frequently seen on the face, hands, or other exposed areas. It usually ranges from three millimeters to less than one centimeter (approximately 1/10 to 1/2 of an inch) in size.

Seborrheic Keratosis: This very common growth is seen more often on elderly people. It has been described as having a "stuck-on" appearance and a waxy feel. It ranges in color from light tan to brown or black. The appearance of this lesion can mimic melanoma. Again, when there is any doubt, it is important to see an expert who can properly evaluate this condition.

Actinic Keratosis: A rough, scaly, sometimes red patch of skin. It is commonly seen on sun-exposed areas, such as the face. It carries a low risk of becoming squamous cell carcinoma.

Blue Nevus: Usually this type of pigmented lesion is less than one centimeter (about ½ inch) and is blue, blue-gray, or blue-black. It usually appears as a single lesion, is uniform in color and regularly-shaped.

Reasons to Remove Common Skin Lesions

Although they are sometimes called "beauty marks," many moles can be physically unattractive. For this and other reasons, you may wish to have a dermatologist surgically remove a normal-appearing mole. The decision to do so depends on a variety of individual factors.

- **Cosmetic Removal**: Many people would rather have a tiny scar than a mole. Sometimes an "ugly" mole has some pre-cancerous cells within it.
- **Irritation**: Moles near a bra strap, belt or on the neck can become irritated. They can sometimes look different after they have been irritated, leading to questions about whether the mole is changing for other reasons.
- **Hidden Moles**: Because self-examination is such an important part of early detection, it may be wise to remove a mole that is difficult to see or monitor. Areas that are often missed are the scalp and the genital area.

Our skin communicates signs of danger when its familiar features change. Surviving melanoma depends upon awareness of our outermost organ and an appreciation of its variations.

CHAPTER 5

Screening for Melanoma

Every spring since 1985, dermatologists around the country have participated in a national skin cancer screening day. At no charge, individuals have the opportunity to be examined by dermatologists. Since the program began, over 600,000 Americans have been examined. In 1991, dermatologists screened approximately 104,000 people, and from that group more than 1,000 suspected melanomas were detected. Most of the melanomas that were found during the screenings were curable.

Epiluminescence Microscopy:
A New Way to Look at Moles

Large melanomas are usually easy for a dermatologist to identify with the naked eye, but smaller early ones are more difficult to assess. Unfortunately, by the time some melanomas become large and easy-to-find, their potential to spread to other parts of the body has increased dramatically. It is for this reason that methods are now being developed to detect early small moles just beginning their malignant changes.

A technique called Epiluminescence Microscopy (ELM) is an important advance in the detection of early melanoma. It allows a doctor to examine the sub-surface of moles not visible to the naked eye. This enhanced view of the interior of a mole may help make diagnoses more accurate. The technique is simple, involving only a drop of mineral oil and a hand-held microscope. The oil, which is applied to a small glass plate and then pressed against the skin, eliminates scattered light off the skin surface and allows a view into the mole. Structures inside the mole, made visible with ELM, provide clues as to whether the mole is malignant or benign.

Dr. Robert Kenet (Dr. Barney Kenet's brother), a board-certified internist and cardiologist with a Ph.D. in electrical engineering, has combined his medical and computer background to create technology that has advanced the uses of ELM. He has spent the last five years developing methods that use computer software and sophisticated cameras to create highly precise digital images of moles.

"We have begun to detect patterns in these images that may eventually enable doctors to detect melanoma in its earliest stage. Today, the only way to definitively diagnose melanoma is to have the tissue surgically removed and analyzed by a pathologist," Dr. Kenet says. His work is leading the way for a future in which a "bloodless biopsy" may be performed with computer images.

"We are now trying to identify patterns and common characteristics within moles that suggest the presence of melanoma. Digital ELM may also help to accurately identify benign moles that mimic melanoma," Dr. Kenet says.

Watching Out For Yourself

Screening by doctors and enhanced imaging techniques are important, but individual self-examination is an inexpensive, safe, and quick way to find suspicious moles early. Everyone should perform a self-examination once a month.

A thorough self-examination should take place in front of a full-length mirror in a well-lit room. A hand-held mirror is the only tool needed. A partner can assist in examining parts of the body that are difficult to see. The illustrations demonstrate how the examination should take place. If you spot a suspicious mole during a self-examination, see a dermatologist promptly for further evaluation.

Watching Out For Each Other

Melanoma adds new meaning to the phrase "You watch my back, I'll watch yours." Husbands, wives, parents, and even friends can do a great service for each other by keeping their eyes open for suspicious moles.

Doctors at the Boston University School of Medicine asked a group of melanoma patients "Who first noticed your melanoma?" Almost one-half of those surveyed said that they did not find the melanoma themselves. It had been spotted by a family member, doctor or someone else. People over the age of 60 were more likely to have a physician discover the melanoma. This should alert adult children to be vigilant in inspecting their parents' skin.

Women Discover Melanoma Sooner Than Men

From childhood, women have been told to be dainty, thin, and smooth-skinned. They have measured themselves against an ideal created by sometimes unrealistic cultural stereotypes. As a result, many women in our society remain preoccupied with their appearance and its enhancement. Still, there are occasions when the concern for appearance can be a key to survival. Consider the case of noted feminist Susan Brownmiller. In an essay on skin, Brownmiller candidly recalls her struggle when she thought she was growing whiskers on her chin. After trying to remove the unwanted hairs herself, she sought the help of a professional. She wrote:

"I furtively visited an electrologist. She peered through a magnifying glass and pronounced her judgement: 'It's a mole.'" Although apparently benign, the mole on Brownmiller's chin had quickly gotten her attention. She concludes wryly, "A mole is a great relief when a woman fears that her drive for success has caused her to sprout whiskers." Susan Brownmiller's anecdote lends credence to the conclusion reached by researchers: Women are more likely than men to examine details of their skin, and thus to find changes on it. They are also more likely to find suspicious moles on their husbands' bodies. By contrast, husbands are less likely to find their own melanomas and very rarely find their wives'. Although this disease strikes both men and women almost equally, women tend to have better survival rates. The authors of the Boston University study noted that this difference has not been easily explained. They do say, however, that self-examination may lead women to find melanoma in its earlier stages, and may possibly explain the better outcomes for females.

Some studies suggest that women tend to have a better prognosis because their melanomas appear on sites of the body that usually have better outcomes. Whether it is because of complex biological differences or not, the vigilance of women surveying their own bodies and their spouse's bodies is a step in the right direction. What some might argue is symptomatic of vanity can in fact be a lifesaving self-awareness.

Losing a Father to Melanoma

Dr. Arthur Rhodes, Professor of Dermatology at the University of Pittsburgh School of Medicine, has been studying moles and melanoma for over 20 years. His most profound experience with the disease, however, occurred at the very beginning of his career. Dr. Rhodes was already an internist

Skin Self Examination

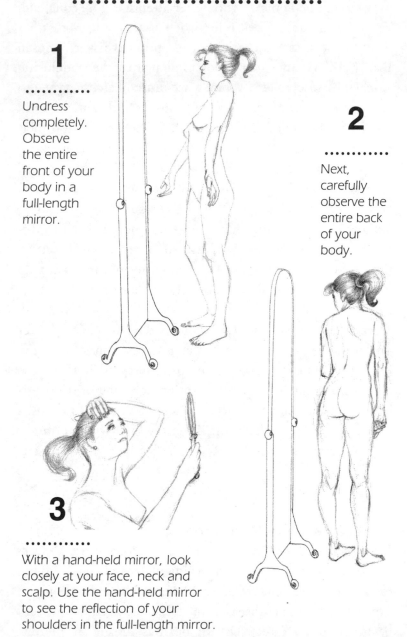

1

Undress completely. Observe the entire front of your body in a full-length mirror.

2

Next, carefully observe the entire back of your body.

3

With a hand-held mirror, look closely at your face, neck and scalp. Use the hand-held mirror to see the reflection of your shoulders in the full-length mirror.

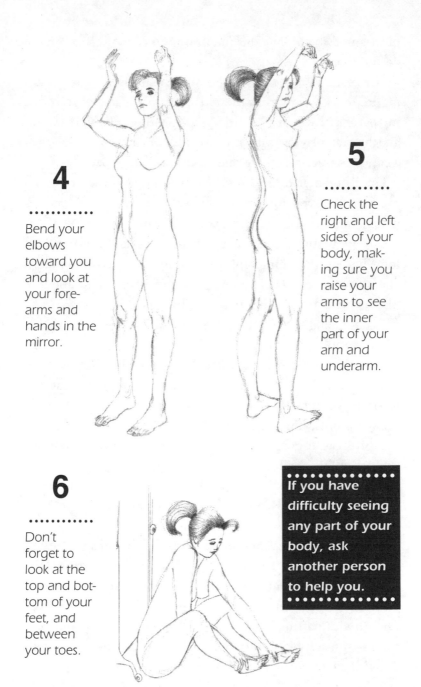

4

Bend your elbows toward you and look at your forearms and hands in the mirror.

5

Check the right and left sides of your body, making sure you raise your arms to see the inner part of your arm and underarm.

6

Don't forget to look at the top and bottom of your feet, and between your toes.

If you have difficulty seeing any part of your body, ask another person to help you.

but wanted to continue his medical training by specializing in dermatology.

"I was in Boston, ready to go into the army for basic training in Texas. On the way there, I went to Philadelphia to visit my parents. I was in the yard with my father. His shirt was off and he was playing with my two kids. From about 15 yards away, I spotted something on my father's left upper back."

Dr. Rhodes had just come from a medical lecture about melanoma given by Dr. Thomas Fitzpatrick at Harvard, which he said was an eye opener because he didn't know much about the disease at the time. "I asked my dad how long he had this thing and he said he had been watching it change for a year. He knew about it, my mom knew about it. She had encouraged him to see a physician."

Recognizing the serious nature of his father's problem, Dr. Rhodes took immediate action. "I brought my father to the dermatologist the next day. I said, 'Is this what I think it is?' and he said, 'Yes.' " His father's lesion was removed the following day. For the next three years, Dr. Rhodes' father had no symptoms, but the disease had already begun to spread. Despite two operations to remove recurring melanoma tumors on his brain, the disease progressed.

"His only request was that he not be in pain. He never complained. He lapsed into a coma and we let him go," Dr. Rhodes recalls.

Sadly, Dr. Rhodes did not discover his father's melanoma until it had spread. In the early 1970s, public education and screening efforts had not begun in earnest. Today increased awareness, early detection and intervention are saving lives. Dr. Rhodes has made a commitment to this cause and continues to teach his students, patients and the general public about the benefits of early detection.

CHAPTER 6

After Identification

Biopsy for Melanoma

If, after careful examination, a doctor suspects that your mole is malignant, a biopsy will be performed. A biopsy is the removal and examination of a tissue sample used to establish a precise diagnosis. Although there are many biopsy techniques for the skin, only two are appropriate for the diagnosis of a suspected malignant melanoma—excisional biopsy and incisional biopsy. Both techniques are usually performed in a doctor's office. Local anesthesia, which is introduced into the skin with a hypodermic needle, numbs the area so that the tissue sample can be removed painlessly. You will, however, be awake during the entire procedure and be able to sense touch or pressure.

Excisional biopsy of a suspected melanoma is the complete removal of the suspicious mole. It is the preferred method of biopsy. A small margin of normal-appearing skin surrounding the mole is also removed.

Incisional biopsy is the removal of a portion of the mole. It can be compared to taking one wedge out of a pie. If the suspicious mole is large or is on a delicate part of your body such as the face, you may have an incisional biopsy. Usually, the darkest part of the lesion or the area that is most raised is removed if possible. This allows for the examination of the most abnormal piece of the mole to determine if further surgery is necessary. If the tissue appears benign under a microscope, a repeat biopsy may have to be performed. If the portion of tissue contains cancer cells, a complete excisional biopsy will be done. Neither an excisional nor an incisional biopsy accelerates the growth or spread of melanoma.

Biopsy techniques that are *not* recommended for the removal of a suspected melanoma include shaving, burning, or curettage (scraping). These procedures are not effective because they may fail to obtain the entire skin sample or destroy part of it during removal. Most importantly, these techniques interfere with the ability to determine the thickness of the melanoma, which is an essential piece of information for treatment and prognosis.

After a suspected mole is removed, it is sent to a laboratory for analysis. An experienced pathologist, preferably a dermatopathologist (a specialist in the microscopic diagnosis of skin disease), examines the tissue sample under a microscope to determine whether it contains malignant cells. If it does, the pathologist will measure the thickness of the melanoma and provide this information to your doctor in a biopsy report. A malignant mole is often referred to as the *primary melanoma* or *primary lesion.*

An accurate analysis of a suspected melanoma is vitally important. In some cases, you may wish to seek out a second opinion. A second opinion does not require additional surgery. The original sample is simply sent to another pathologist who prepares a second report. You should consider obtaining a second opinion if your primary doctor recommends additional treatment based on the original report.

Re-excision of the Surgical Site

If the skin sample is malignant, additional surgery may be necessary to remove some of the normal-appearing skin that surrounded the site of the primary melanoma. This procedure can usually be performed in a doctor's office with local anesthesia, depending on the size and thickness of the mole.

Removal of a malignant melanoma should be performed by a competent professional. A dermatologist is qualified to remove a primary melanoma, as is a general surgeon, a plastic surgeon or a surgical oncologist, a surgeon who is specially trained in the removal of tumors.

One of the major concerns in battling malignant melanoma is the removal of both the mole and a sufficient border of normal skin around it. The diameter of the area to be removed is typically determined by the thickness of the mole, its location and appearance. The surrounding healthy skin is removed to eliminate any melanoma cells that may have migrated out from the tumor. Such "damage control" may reduce the risk that the melanoma will spread to other parts of the body. In the past, doctors tended to remove a wide area of healthy tissue surrounding a melanoma, which in some instances resulted in disfigurement or required skin grafting. In recent years, studies have shown that a more conservative approach, removing a smaller area of healthy skin, is adequate. Generally speaking, the thicker the melanoma, the wider the area around it that will be excised.

The complete surgical removal of a melanoma is essential. All of the detectable tumor must be removed from the skin so that the chance for the spread of malignant cells is reduced.

Preventing the Return of Melanoma

Is there anything that you can do to keep melanoma from returning after it has been surgically removed? Today there is no recommended treatment for preventing the recurrence of melanoma. Good nutrition, regular exercise and avoiding sunburns may help to keep your immune system healthy. A positive attitude may also work to your benefit, according to some recent studies.

Adjuvant therapy is the use of anti-cancer or other drugs to delay or prevent the return of cancer after it has been surgically removed. Vaccines and other immunologic treatments are being tested on an experimental basis to determine whether they will work to prevent a recurrence. A discussion of experimental therapy is provided in Chapter 12.

Treatment of Scars After Melanoma Excision

The size of the wound created by surgical removal of the melanoma and surrounding skin depends on the size and thickness of the primary melanoma. Usually, a small wound is closed with stitches, which generally results in a small straight scar. In some areas, the scar can spread slightly in the center, especially if the surgery was performed on the back or chest.

If the wound is large and cannot be closed with stitches, reconstructive surgery may be necessary. Doctors use skin flaps and grafts to cover a wound created by a large excision. A skin flap involves taking healthy skin adjacent to the wound and pulling it over the surgical site. A graft, on the other hand, is the complete removal of a section of skin from another part of the body and its transplantation onto the excision site. Extensive surgical repair is sometimes delayed for a year, if possible, so that the wound can be observed in its natural state for any signs of a recurrence.

Wounds heal better if you are in good health. Vitamins A, C, and E help the healing process. Also, avoiding alcohol and tobacco can go a long way to improve healing. Skin flaps and grafts heal poorly in smokers, so smoking should be avoided, especially during the days before and after surgery.

The surgical removal of a melanoma in its earliest stage is

the equivalent of a cure. This cure has minimal side effects and its cost is relatively low. As the disease progresses, its treatment becomes increasingly harsh and decreasingly effective. If we remain vigilant in our efforts at early detection, someday a simple surgical procedure may be the only treatment we need to cure melanoma.

CHAPTER 7

Staging of Melanoma

As a professional football player for the Green Bay Packers for 14 years, Forrest Gregg's accomplishments were measured by impressive statistics. Gregg played in 188 consecutive games, participating in six NFL championship games. He was considered the power of the Packers' offensive line, making All-Pro eight times and playing in the Pro-Bowl nine times. He led Green Bay to Super Bowl titles in 1966 and 1967. Following his brilliant career as a player, Gregg became a leader on the sidelines. He became head coach of the Cleveland Browns in 1975 and a year later was named NFL Coach of the Year.

In that same year, shortly before being inducted into the Pro-Football Hall of Fame, Gregg, then 42 years old, was diagnosed with melanoma. From that point on, his life centered around statistics of a different sort.

Gregg remembers how the birthmark on his thigh had changed over the years before he had it examined. "It began to change colors a bit, but I didn't think much about it because it had always been there." Gradually, the mark became dark and irregular, and in 1976, when he put on a bathing suit while on vacation, he noticed that the mole was becoming bumpy. He realized then that he needed medical attention, and called a dermatologist. Gregg knew he had no time to waste, and had the changing mole biopsied. "We got our ducks in line," he says. "My mole was removed and it was confirmed to be malignant."

The news that followed was no better. The melanoma on Gregg's thigh was thick enough to indicate that the cancer might have spread. For the first time in his life, Gregg's statistics were dismal. "They gave me a 50-50 chance to live to five years," he says. Surgery was performed on Gregg's lymph nodes, and while no additional tumors were found, his prognosis, according to standardized statistics for melanoma, remained unchanged. Five years came and went, a decade and then 15 years, without any further evidence of cancer. As each year passes, Gregg, who is now working as athletic director of Southern Methodist University, feels that he is a true winner. "Today, I don't take anything for granted," he says.

At the time of Gregg's diagnosis, researchers were just beginning to understand how the thickness of a melanoma correlates with survival. While the news may not always be good, many melanoma patients want to know the extent of their disease and their chance of survival in order to plan their lives with realistic expectations.

One 25-year-old man, David, recalls that after surgery for what turned out to be a recurrence of melanoma, he appreciated his doctor's candor regarding his prognosis.

"Because I'm the kind of guy who doesn't like to be surprised, my doctor sat down and told me what was happening, what the situation was, and what I could expect. He told me that I had a 40 percent chance of being alive in three years, which stuck in my mind. He wasn't morbid about it, just up-front. He didn't say, 'This is what's going to happen to you,' only, 'This is what you have, these are our dealings with it so far, and these are your statistics.' That was the way I wanted to hear it."

For David, what mattered most was obtaining the information and proceeding from there. For those who want to know more about their disease and its associated survival rate, staging is a starting point.

What is Staging?
Staging provides information about prognosis, the probable outcome of a disease. Staging allows physicians to communicate with each other and their patients by using a common criteria for assessing the extent of the illness. It helps a patient understand what the future probably holds, and guides him or her in making informed decisions about treatment options and their associated risks.

Staging helps an individual and his or her family make personal decisions. If the disease is advanced, a person may wish to set short-term goals. In other instances, when the disease is detected and treated at an early stage, an individual can plan his or her life and look to the future with optimism and peace of mind.

As with much medical information, the survival statistics associated with staging can be cold and impersonal. They generalize about groups of patients based on average survival and cannot take into account a multitude of variables such as motivation, support from family and friends, nutrition, and stress levels, all of which may have an impact on a cancer patient's survival. There is no factoring in the statistical system for faith and hope, the bedrock of emotional therapy for someone faced with a life-threatening disease.

Melanoma can behave in unpredictable ways. In some rare cases, it can disappear spontaneously. It is not uncommon for a patient with poor prognostic signs to survive for years, or in seemingly early cases for the disease to progress rapidly. Bearing all this in mind, these staging figures are presented as the most comprehensive statistics available to date in the imperfect world of science.

Vertical and Horizontal Growth

Melanoma grows in two ways. There is a horizontal growth phase, during which it spreads across the surface of the skin. At a later point, the melanoma may begin to grow vertically, invading into the deeper layers of the skin. This phase of growth is dangerous because the melanoma then has a chance to enter the blood and lymphatic vessels and eventually spread to the lymph nodes and other parts of the body.

Staging Systems

There are two types of staging—microstaging and clinical staging—which measure melanoma and provide a system for predicting prognosis.

Microstaging

Microstaging is the measurement of melanoma with the use of a microscope after the melanoma has been surgically removed. Microstaging measures the thickness of the tumor and the level of skin that it has invaded. Most experts agree that the thickness of a melanoma is the single most important predictor for survival in cases where there is no evidence of spread to other parts of the body.

Tumor Thickness and Survival

Dr. Alexander Breslow of George Washington University first grouped melanoma by thickness and corresponding rates of survival in the early 1970s. In the chart below, tumor thickness predicts the statistical likelihood of five-year survival for patients with primary tumors but no other signs of melanoma. Under the standardized Breslow system, pathologists measure melanomas in millimeters from top to bottom.

Breslow Microstaging for Melanoma

Thickness in millimeters/inches	5-Year Survival Rate
Less than or equal to 0.75 mm(about 1/32 inch)	96%
0.76-1.49 mm(about 1/32 to 1/16 inch)	87%
1.5-2.49 mm (about 1/16 to 1/11 inch)	75%
2.50-3.99 mm(about 1/11 to 1/8 inch)	66%
Greater than or equal to 4.0 mm(about 1/8 inch)	47%

These statistics illustrate that millimeters can have a significant impact on survival.

Clark's Levels

The second microstaging method is called "Clark's Levels of Invasion." Developed by Dr. Wallace Clark, Jr. at the University of Pennsylvania Medical School in 1969, this measuring system characterizes the relationship between deeper levels of invasion into the skin and poorer prognosis. Clark's Levels do not measure melanoma in millimeters, but rather describe into which layer of the skin the melanoma has penetrated. As each layer is invaded, there is a greater likelihood that the malignant cells may have spread. Because of individual variations in skin thickness, Clark's Levels can sometimes provide a different prognosis than Breslow thickness. Although Clark's Levels are considered significant, the actual thickness of the tumor remains the most relevant factor for prognosis in early melanoma.

Clark's Levels of Invasion

Level I: tumor cells confined to the epidermis, the top layer of the skin. This is also known as melanoma *in situ*.

Level II: tumor cells penetrate into the papillary dermis, the uppermost portion of the dermis, the second layer of the skin.

Level III: tumor cells completely fill the papillary dermis, but do not enter the reticular dermis, the deep portion of the dermis

Level IV: tumor cells enter the reticular dermis

Level V: tumor cells fill the dermis and enter the subcutaneous fat.

Survival rates decrease with each level of invasion. The thicker the growth, the greater the likelihood that malignant cells have spread to other parts of the body. Conversely, thinner tumors are more likely to have a favorable prognosis.

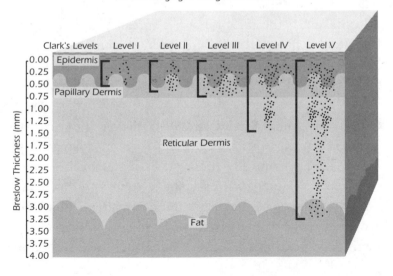

BRESLOW THICKNESS AND CLARK'S LEVELS
for Microstaging of Malignant Melanoma

Over 90 percent of patients with a thin invasive melanoma—less than one millimeter (about 1/25 of an inch), a little thicker than your thumbnail—will have long-term, disease-free survival if the lesion is completely removed.

Clinical Staging

Clinical staging uses a doctor's physical examination of the patient, as well as tests such as x-rays, to measure the extent of cancer. Standard clinical staging for all types of cancer uses three main categories: Local Disease (Stage I); Regional Metastasis (Stage II); and Distant Metastasis (Stage III). Stage I is sometimes referred to as (T) for tumor, Stage II as (N) for node and Stage III as (M) for metastasis.

For melanoma, clinical staging has been categorized this way:

Stage I means that the melanoma is confined to its original site. There is no sign of spread to the lymph nodes or other organs.

Stage II indicates that melanoma has spread to the lymph nodes. The prognosis of Stage II is, in many cases, dependent upon the number of lymph nodes containing cancer cells as well as the size of the tumors within them.

In Stage III, the melanoma has spread to other organs. Prognosis in Stage III is influenced by the number and type of organs affected by the cancer and whether or not the tumors in other parts of the body can be surgically removed.

Combining Clinical Staging and Microstaging

Clinical staging was developed before microstaging for melanoma. Lumping all patients with Stage I melanoma into one group fails to take into account significant differences in survival predicted by the tumor thickness or level of invasion provided under the microstaging systems. Using clinical staging alone to evaluate melanoma therefore sometimes presents an inaccurate prognostic picture for a patient with Stage I disease. Since up to 85% of all melanoma patients are diagnosed with Stage I disease, a new system, combining microstaging and clinical staging information was needed.

In 1988, The American Joint Committee on Cancer (A.J.C.C.) and the Union Internationale Contre le Cancer (U.I.C.C.) Staging System was developed and is now used by many doctors.

The A.J.C.C./U.I.C.C. Staging System

STAGE	CRITERIA
IA	Primary melanoma less than or equal to 0.75 mm thick (about 1/32 of an inch) and/or Clark's Level II; no sign of tumors in the nodes or any other organ.
IB	Primary melanoma 0.76 to 1.5 mm thick (about 1/32 to 1/16 of an inch) and/or Clark's Level III; no sign of tumors in the nodes or other organ.
IIA	Primary melanoma 1.51 to 4 mm thick (about 1/16 to 1/8 of an inch) and/or Clark's Level IV; no signs of tumors in the nodes or other organs.
IIB	Primary melanoma greater than 4 mm thick (about 1/8 of an inch) and/or Clark's Level V; no signs of tumors in the nodes or any other organs.
III	Spread to the regional lymph nodes and/or in-transit metastatic tumors (tumors that have spread from the primary melanoma and are travelling toward the lymph nodes).
IV	Spread to distant parts of the body.

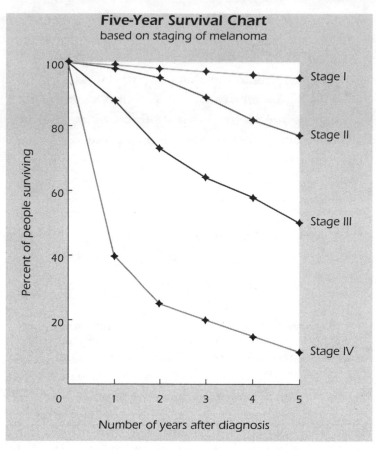

Five-Year Survival Chart
based on staging of melanoma

Percent of people surviving

Stage I
Stage II
Stage III
Stage IV

Number of years after diagnosis

Adapted from: Beahrs, Oliver H., Manual for Staging of Cancer, *fourth edition. Philadelphia: J.B. Lippincott, 1992.*

The four stages have been analyzed in terms of patient survival over a five-year period. As the stage increases, the chance for survival declines.

Tests to Determine Clinical Staging

A complete physical examination, including palpation of the lymph nodes, liver and spleen for evidence of tumors, is required in order to obtain an accurate assessment of the clinical stage. Your physician will also need to obtain a complete medical history. Your entire skin surface should be inspected to determine if there are any other suspicious moles or signs that the melanoma has spread. Your doctor may use a Wood's Lamp to examine the skin surface. This device emits longwave ultraviolet "black" light that helps the doctor detect changes on the skin. This exam is conducted with the overhead lighting turned off.

Generally speaking, a person with Clinical Stage I melanoma usually will need a baseline chest X-ray and a blood test. The presence of any swelling in the lymph nodes may require a biopsy of the nodes.

The National Institutes of Health recently issued a statement that laboratory tests or scans such as a CT-Scan, MRI or a nuclear scan are only warranted for those patients who have physical symptoms in addition to the primary melanoma. Thus, if you have any symptoms such as persistent headaches, pain, or dizziness, for example, you should bring them to your doctor's attention.

Other Prognostic Factors

In addition to tumor thickness, other characteristics of the primary melanoma may affect your prognosis. How these factors influence survival is still poorly understood.

Ulceration: A primary melanoma may be ulcerated, meaning that the lesion resembles an open sore accompanied by the erosion of tissue. Ulceration is associated with a poorer prognosis.

Location of the Primary Melanoma on the Body: Patients with melanomas on their arms or legs (excluding hands, feet and nails) may have a better overall survival rate than patients whose primary melanoma appears on the trunk, head or neck.

Age: Advanced age is usually associated with a poorer prognosis.

Sex: Several studies indicate that women have a better rate of survival than men. However, these findings have been questioned because melanoma in women usually appears on the extremities and is diagnosed when the tumor is thin, and less ulcerated.

Other variables include measurement of cell activity, microscopic tumors near the original melanoma, and a phenomenon known as regression, which is the disappearance of pigment in the primary melanoma. Whether or not regression indicates a poorer prognosis has not been fully determined.

Tumor Volume

Tumor volume is defined as the mass of the tumor, not just its thickness. Physicians at New York University School of Medicine have challenged the idea that thickness is the best predictor of survival. If the mass of the primary tumor is so great that it requires an additional blood supply, new blood vessels may form. According to studies done by N.Y.U.'s Dr. R. J. Friedman, the lethal nature of melanoma is related to its capacity to stimulate the formation of new tumor-associated blood vessels under the skin. These new vessels may be more easily penetrated by melanoma cancer cells than normal blood vessels, thus increasing the chance for spread of melanoma through the bloodstream.

This type of tumor measurement is still being investigated. It is not used on a regular basis, partly because it is somewhat difficult to calculate. Nevertheless, the tumor volume analysis may be an important new method of determining prognosis.

The Intangibles

Unlike the scientific criteria discussed above, many other factors that may influence survival cannot be measured or calculated, or even seen. Faith, optimism and a feeling of control enhance our lives. They become even more important when we are seriously ill.

Melanoma, more than many types of cancer, seems to be influenced by the complex workings of our immune system. Recent studies have shown that there may be a relationship between the survival of a melanoma patient and his or her attitude at the onset of the disease. These findings suggest that there are mysteries and miracles within us that may defy the numbers. Until the answers to these questions are found, melanoma patients need to meet the challenges posed by their illness with a delicate combination of realism and hope. Staging methods supply a realistic piece of the puzzle; optimism provides another critical component.

CHAPTER 8

Choosing Your Doctor

A Team of Specialists With a Single Goal

Different stages of melanoma call for different types of treatment and, as a result, different types of doctors.

For the removal of a suspected primary melanoma, you will need to see a dermatologist and, possibly, a general or plastic surgeon. Your dermatologist will also rely on the opinion of a dermatopathologist.

Your dermatologist will identify suspected melanomas, perform biopsies as needed and (if necessary) remove a melanoma surgically. The dermatologist's role is also to periodically examine your skin for signs of suspicious changes. A general or plastic surgeon may be needed to complete the removal of the melanoma and a small amount of skin surrounding it.

A doctor whom you will probably never meet, but who will play a crucial role in your diagnosis, is the dermatopathologist. This specialist is an expert in the microscopic diagnosis of skin disorders, and is the most qualified type of physician to determine whether your skin sample contains melanoma cells. As opposed to a general pathologist who looks at many types of tissue samples, a dermatopathologist deals exclusively with disorders of the skin. If your biopsy was read by a general pathologist, consider obtaining a second opinion from a dermatopathologist.

If there is a possibility that the melanoma has spread to other parts of your body, your primary care doctor or dermatologist may refer you to a medical oncologist—a doctor who specializes in the treatment of cancer with chemotherapy. You may also need to see a surgeon again, preferably a surgical oncologist and one experienced in dealing with melanoma.

If you have been diagnosed with a thick primary melanoma, but have limited or no evidence of spread to other parts of the body, you may be referred to a center where experimental adjuvant therapy trials are offered. This type of therapy is aimed at preventing the recurrence of cancer after all evidence of it has been surgically removed.

Most likely, your primary doctor knows the specialist and is satisfied that he or she is capable. If you are not sure whether your referring doctor knows the specialist, feel free to ask and also to discuss why this particular doctor may be right for you.

The recommendation of a personal physician, friend, or cancer patient may be your best resource, especially if the person knows you well and understands your personal needs. Your local hospital's physician referral service can also recommend a doctor who specializes in the care of patients with cancer, or possibly one experienced in melanoma in particular. The National Cancer Institute and the American Cancer Society as well as your local county medical society are also good places to inquire about specialists in your area.

If you have private health insurance, either through your employer or a policy that you purchased on your own, you will probably be able to select your physician based on the recommendations described above. If you are insured through an H.M.O. or other managed health care organization, your choice may be limited to those physicians participating in this group.

What To Look For in a Doctor

Skill and experience are vital, but you may be interested in a doctor with other qualities as well. Some patients don't care if they like their doctor as long as he or she helps them to get better. These people may seek out a doctor with the best credentials and a well-regarded reputation. Others prefer a specific personality. Every patient looks for something different: a good listener, an aggressive fighter, someone with similar religious beliefs, even someone of the same or opposite sex.

You should understand that a doctor cannot be all things. He or she can provide guidance and outline treatment options, but ultimately the decisions about your care are your own. A doctor can be supportive and caring, but cannot be a substitute for family or friends. A doctor's role is to manage your medical care with competency and compassion. Together you are players on the same team with the same goals.

As you begin to make a choice, there are some things to keep in mind. Any doctor should be willing to discuss the following matters with you, and should be obliging if you desire a second opinion, or even a third, about your diagnosis or treatment.

Below are some questions you might consider asking your prospective doctor:

- **Is the oncologist board certified?** Within the field of oncology, there are various sub-specialties. Medical oncologists administer chemotherapy; radiation oncologists use radiation to shrink tumors; surgical oncologists specialize in removing tumors.

  A *board certified* designation means that the physician, after completion of specialized training, has passed an examination given by specialists in the field. Board certification in medical oncology is relatively new, so some older doctors may not be board certified. However, they may be qualified to treat you based on their years of experience. Since there is no board of surgical oncology, it is best to find a board certified general surgeon who has experience in the removal of melanoma tumors.

- **How much experience does the doctor have in treating melanoma?** Because melanoma is difficult to treat in its advanced stages and is a relatively uncommon cancer, you want an oncologist with experience in treating it.
- **Is the doctor on the staff of a medical school-affiliated hospital?** An affiliation with a medical school or university hospital generally demonstrates that the doctor has an interest in ongoing education within his field. It may also mean, but not necessarily guarantee, that he or she is exposed to the latest developments in treatment. And affiliation implies the support and acceptance of colleagues within a medical community.
- **Is the doctor well informed about experimental therapy?** The treatment options for melanoma are changing rapidly. Many of the newer ones are experimental. If you are interested in exploring the possibility of experimental therapies, you should consider an oncologist who is familiar with or involved in clinical trials in which you could participate. If your doctor is not affiliated with an institution offering experimental treatment, he or she should be familiar with experimental trials being offered in your region of the country.

Further Questions

Besides asking the doctor questions, you, as a patient, need to make decisions based on your feelings and observations about the doctor and his or her staff:

- **Is the doctor ready to answer all of your questions, and willing to admit that he or she doesn't know some of the answers?** Will the doctor try to find out what you need to know?

- **Is the doctor taking the necessary time to answer your questions and address your concerns?** Your doctor should try to answer all of your questions. He or she should communicate with you at each appointment. To save time and help you remember, try to think of your questions and write them down before each visit. Remember that effective communication is a two-way street. Listen carefully to your doctor's answers. Take notes if you need to. Listening to information about your own disease, especially if the condition is serious, is difficult. Even the most sophisticated person can misinterpret or miss information entirely in those circumstances. A friend or family member can be helpful by providing an extra set of ears.

- **Does the doctor answer questions in a clear and understandable manner that is compatible with your level of comprehension?**

- **Does the doctor have office hours that suit your schedule?**

- **Is the doctor's staff courteous, compassionate and discreet?** Is it well-organized with an efficient system for taking your calls and making appointments?

Doctor, Patient, Family

Cancer is a disease that affects not only the patient, but the patient's family as well. Family support is a critical part of a person's sense of well-being, yet sometimes family members have different opinions about the right kind of care for the patient. The patient's wishes regarding treatment should never go unheard over the clamor of well-meaning relatives whose input is based on their own feelings.

One oncologist recalls an incident in which the husband and daughter of a melanoma patient called him and requested that he discuss hospice care with the patient because of her advanced condition. The doctor reluctantly complied and broached the subject with his patient. "I told her that her chance of responding to the therapy was about ten percent. I said she might want to go to a hospice." He recalls the woman's reaction: "Why would you say something like that to me? I chose you because I believed you would fight with me until the end." In fact, that had always been the doctor's intention. That patient's family imposed their desires, however well-meaning, into the delicate balance of the doctor-patient relationship.

Deciding to Change Doctors

Choosing a doctor for a serious disease is a difficult decision; changing doctors is perhaps an even harder one. In Anatole Broyard's book describing his battle with prostate cancer, he writes about his growing unease with his oncologist. He realized that his feelings about his doctor were, in part, irrational, but believed that his decision did not need to be based entirely on hard facts. He writes:

> What turned me against him was what I saw as a lack of style or magic. I realized that I wanted my doctor to have magic as well as medical ability. It was like having a lucky doctor. I've described all this—a patient's madness—to show how irrational such transactions are, how far removed from any notion of dispassionate objectivity. To be sick is already to be disordered in your mind as well. Still, this does not necessarily mean that I was wrong to want to change doc-

tors: I was simply listening to my unconscious telling me what I needed. I feel that my absurdity is part of myself. I have to accommodate it. I wanted a doctor who would answer to my absurdity and triumph over it.

Patients change doctors for any number of reasons, ranging from an inconvenient office location to serious difficulties in patient-doctor interaction. Other people change based on a "gut reaction" as described by Broyard. Throughout the patient-doctor relationship, it is vital that you communicate your feelings of discomfort or unhappiness. Many times the situation can be greatly improved by simply voicing your concerns. Other times, the decision to change is right.

In 1988, a young woman was diagnosed with a recurrence of melanoma in her lung and abdomen. She recalls the reaction of her physicians at a major university hospital. "My oncologists told me to go home and wait. They told me that if the pain got too bad, they would give me painkillers," she says, her voice still resonant with disbelief and anger. "In looking back, I think it's strange to tell someone who's 25 to give up."

Unwilling to accept her doctors' death sentence, she went to the National Institutes of Health in Bethesda, Maryland, for experimental therapy. She was pleased with the attitudes of her new doctors. "When I went to NIH everyone said, 'We can deal with this. You're not hopeless.'"

Despite serious side effects, the treatment shrank the tumors and further treatments have reduced them even more. Although she is not technically "cured," she feels much better both physically and emotionally than she did when her first set of doctors sent her home. She is working full-time and leading an active life. So while her doctors might have been ready to give up hope, she was not.

Ginny, a social worker and family therapist, was faced with a recurrence of melanoma in her lymph nodes four years after a primary tumor was removed from her back. After the removal of her nodes, she was referred to an oncologist recommended by her surgeon. Ginny has a full rich laugh, and it is difficult to miss the fact that she is an upbeat person with a remarkable sense of humor, despite her serious condition. She describes her first oncologist this way: "She was so remote, impersonal. She didn't inspire confidence. She was just not emotionally available."

Ginny also remembers other things that simply did not satisfy her about the doctor. "The staff never smiled when I came for visits," she recalls. "I didn't feel welcome. Even the decorating in the office was ugly."

Although she stayed with her oncologist for a while, she eventually met another woman who had also been a patient of this doctor and reinforced Ginny's feelings. After that encounter, despite no further signs of melanoma, Ginny knew it was time to change. "Don't wait for a crisis to happen before you change doctors," she advises. Through a patient's recommendation, she found a new oncologist who has a "human quality" that makes Ginny feel very comfortable. Ginny also suggests that any melanoma patient faced with finding an oncologist get feedback from people who have been through this ordeal and can recommend a doctor from their own experience.

Another patient, Don Gorelick, 44, of Apple Valley, California, has devoted much of his life to helping others. In 1988, when Don was diagnosed with advanced melanoma, he utilized his background as an educator and consumer advocate to find out which doctor and treatment plan would work best for him. Don understood that his disease was serious, and he wanted a physician who could offer him some degree of hope.

Don was very disappointed by the attitude of his first two doctors. One of them, Don recalls, "didn't tell me—but told my wife—that I had about 12 months to live. He never talked about alternative medicine, diet or other options, which were very important to me and my family. Another doctor said that I had about as much chance of being cured as of winning the lottery.

"That's not the right way to talk to someone faced with a serious disease," Don continues. "He should tell me that I have a difficult cancer, but he should say it in language that will not devastate me to the point that I don't even want to get off my chair and try anymore."

When his cancer re-appeared several years later, Don knew what kind of doctor he needed. He wanted someone who would try as hard as he did, someone who could offer him some hope. He found such a doctor and entered into an experimental vaccine program. Today, Don is doing well, and he is happy that he decided to follow his own instincts.

The diagnosis of cancer, particularly advanced cancer, can often leave an individual feeling that life is out of control, that he or she has been betrayed by his or her own body. Finding the right doctor and establishing a relationship based on trust, confidence, and common goals can help you feel that you have regained some sense of control. It is an essential and empowering element for improving the quality of life in the face of a serious disease.

CHAPTER 9

When Melanoma Spreads to the Lymph Nodes

The appearance of melanoma in the lymph nodes is frequently one of the first signs that the disease has spread from the original melanoma. In many cases, melanoma that is evident in the lymph nodes requires surgical removal of those nodes. This is called *lymph node dissection*.

The Lymphatic System

The lymphatic system comprises a clear fluid called *lymph*, *lymph vessels*, and *lymph nodes*. Lymph fluid circulates through the body, removing bacteria, viruses, waste products, and excess fluid. The pathways that drain this fluid from the body and direct it into the node are called lymph vessels. A lymph node is a soft, oval-shaped, gray-white structure approximately the size of a kidney bean. Lymph nodes exist in the neck, underarm, and groin, and in fact, throughout the entire body. Lymph nodes are attached to lymph vessels which have numerous connections with the bloodstream. Eventually all of the lymph fluid drains from the lymphatic system back into the bloodstream.

The lymph nodes function as an essential part of the immune system. When the immune system detects an invading organism a complicated process begins which may cause the nodes to enlarge or become tender. This is part of the normal functioning of the immune system. For example, when you have a sore throat, the lymph nodes in your neck can become large and tender. Lymph nodes may also become enlarged if cancer cells travel to the nodes and multiply within them. A node that is invaded by cancer cells is usually firm and painless. The only way to positively determine that a swollen node is harboring cancer cells is by removing it and examining it under the microscope.

Why do melanoma cells appear so often in the lymph nodes? As a melanoma grows down through the layers of the skin, it can penetrate small lymph vessels and travel via lymph fluid to the nodes. The malignant cells in the nodes can multiply and form an enlarging tumor mass within the node.

Cells from a malignant melanoma on the leg usually drain to the lymph region in the groin, known as the *inguinal* region. Cells from a malignant melanoma on the arm tend to drain to the lymph nodes in the underarm, or *axilla*. In certain instances, it is difficult to predict into which nodal region the malignant cells are likely to drain. For example, melanomas on the head and neck and melanomas on the trunk can drain into one or several lymph node areas. Cells from a malignant melanoma on the arm or leg are more likely to have a predictable pathway to a nearby lymph node region.

If you have been diagnosed with melanoma, you should immediately bring any swelling of your lymph nodes to your doctor's attention.

Lymph Node Dissection

Lymph node dissection refers to the surgical removal of a group of lymph nodes. There are two types of lymph node dissections: *therapeutic dissection*, also known as late dissection, and *elective dissection*, also known as prophylactic or early dissection.

Therapeutic Lymph Node Dissection

If you have been diagnosed with melanoma, your physician will periodically examine your lymph nodes for the presence of any growth in those areas. If your doctor suspects that the growth in your nodes is malignant, he or she may perform a biopsy of the node, which is the surgical removal of the infected node. In other situations you may have a fine needle aspiration—the removal of fluid and/or tissue through a needle inserted into the node. In both situations, the tissue sample will be sent to the laboratory for analysis to determine if there are malignant cells present.

If the node is malignant, you will most likely undergo surgery to have the rest of the nodes in that region removed, because they may also be diseased. This procedure is called therapeutic lymph node dissection, or late lymph node dissection. The goal of a therapeutic lymph node dissection is to cure or control the spread of melanoma evident in the nodes, or to alleviate symptoms associated with the presence of the tumor, such as pain, swelling or limited movement.

"The standard practice is that if the nodes are palpable [can be felt], they should be taken out. This is a good procedure for controlling the growth of the tumor," says Dr. Alan Houghton, a melanoma expert at Memorial-Sloan Kettering Cancer Center in New York.

In general, the fewer the number of lymph nodes harboring malignant cells and the smaller their size, the better the prognosis.

Elective Lymph Node Dissection

No one wants to have surgery unnecessarily, but almost everybody would agree to have surgery to save his or her life. This basic premise underlies a major controversy in the treatment of melanoma—*elective lymph node dissection* (ELND). Elective lymph node dissection is the removal of lymph nodes before any tumors can be felt within them. The question is: "Does it save lives to remove normal-feeling nodes for certain patients who run a high risk of having some microscopic malignant cells in those nodes?" If the answer to this question is "yes," then elective lymph node dissection is an important surgical procedure that can save lives. If the answer is "no," then elective lymph node dissections are of no value; they merely place a patient at risk for complications of surgery which has no benefit. Today, we don't have a simple "yes" or "no" answer to this question.

In some ways, the controversy over elective lymph node dissection is like the debate concerning the removal of a women's breast and lymph nodes when a malignant tumor in her breast is discovered (rather than just removing the tumor). The goal is to do whatever is necessary to ensure that all of the cancer cells are removed from the body, but at the same time to avoid needless surgery.

The rationale for elective lymph node dissection is based on the theory that melanoma cells often spread sequentially from the primary melanoma tumor to the regional lymph nodes and then to distant sites of the body. Melanoma cells can also spread to distant lymph nodes. For example, a primary melanoma on the arm can spread to the lymph nodes in the groin. In that situation, the spread is considered to be distant or metastatic.

Removing lymph nodes results in the surgical eradication of microscopic tumors within them. If a lymph node feels normal, however, there is no way to know before surgery whether it in fact contains malignant cells. This can only be determined after the nodes are removed and looked at under a microscope. A lymph node biopsy would only sample a single suspicious node, and this may not provide a complete assessment for the presence of malignant cells in other nodes in that lymph node region. A lymph node dissection, on the other hand, is the removal of all the nodes in a region. Removing the nodes that contain microscopic tumors may halt the spread of the disease or even cure it, according to some doctors.

Only certain types of patients are considered for elective lymph node dissection. They are 1) patients whose melanoma has a clear-cut pathway to the regional lymph nodes (such as melanoma on the arm or leg) and 2) patients who are likely to have melanoma cells in his or her lymph node region but not in any other part of the body. Whether a patient is likely to have melanoma cells within those nodes is determined by the thickness of the original melanoma tumor at the time of diagnosis. After studying thousands of melanoma patients, some doctors think that patients who may benefit from ELND are those with intermediate thickness melanoma (one to four millimeters thick or about 1/25 to 1/8 of an inch). This is because an intermediate thickness melanoma has a 60 percent risk of spreading to the lymph nodes, but a much lower risk of spreading to other parts of the body. For patients with thinner melanomas (less than one millimeter), an elective lymph node dissection is not recommended since a thin melanoma that has been promptly removed will usually not spread to the lymph nodes or any other parts of the body. If the original melanoma was thicker than four millimeters at the time of diagnosis, elective lymph node dissection is not recommended because there is a greater than 70 percent risk that the melanoma has already spread beyond the lymph nodes to other parts of the body. In this situation, removal of the nodes will probably not increase survival significantly. Original tumor thickness is the major factor in determining whether elective lymph node dissection is warranted, but other criteria such as age and the site of the original melanoma are important elements as well.

Those surgeons who advocate elective lymph node dissection argue that the advantage of the procedure is an increased chance of a cure in selected patients. By waiting until the nodes are large enough to be felt, they believe, the chance for a cure decreases because malignant tumors may have already spread to other parts of the body. Doctors at Southern Methodist University who studied over 1300 patients found that those with intermediate thickness melanoma who underwent ELND had improved survival rates compared to those who did not have the surgery.

Other medical experts argue that elective lymph node dissection does not improve survival and merely exposes people to unnecessary surgical risks. Studies conducted by the World Health Organization Melanoma Group and doctors at the Mayo Clinic found that patients undergoing elective lymph node dissection did not live longer than other patients who did not undergo the procedure. Their research indicated that in some cases malignant cells may travel to other parts of the body first before reaching the lymph nodes. When cancer cells bypass the regional lymph nodes and form tumors in other parts of the body first, this is known as *skip metastasis*. In situations where skip metastasis occurs, elective lymph node dissection would be of no benefit to the patient.

Lymphatic Mapping

Is there a way to predict whether there are microscopic cancer cells in a lymph node region without major surgery? Dr. Donald Morton, a melanoma expert at the John Wayne Cancer Center in Santa Monica, California has developed a technique called *lymphatic mapping* which he hopes will identify those patients who will benefit from elective lymph node dissection and spare others from needless surgery.

During the first phase of this procedure, a blue dye is injected into the site of the primary melanoma. If the sentinel node (the first node into which the melanoma cells are likely to travel) picks up the dye, that node is then removed and examined for the presence of cancer. If it contains malignant cells, then the remainder of the lymph nodes in that region will be removed. If the sentinel node does not contain malignant cells, it is unlikely that melanoma is present in neighboring lymph nodes, according to Dr. Morton's theory. Dr. Morton hopes that as this procedure is studied further, it will allow for more accurate assessment of the extent of the disease and help to reserve surgery for those who are most likely to benefit from it.

Side Effects of Lymph Node Dissection

Some of the short-term risks associated with lymph node dissection include wound infection, fluid collection at the site of the wound, and nerve dysfunction. Most of these problems are not permanent, but they may require some patients to have prolonged hospital stays. Other more long-term risks include pain and *lymphedema*.

Lymphedema is the swelling of a body part, often an arm or leg, due to the accumulation of lymphatic fluid from the disruption of the lymphatic system after surgery. For some people, this is a temporary condition that improves with time and is alleviated with certain forms of exercise. For others, especially those who had inguinal lymph node (groin area) dissection, the condition can last longer.

Paul, an engineer, was diagnosed with melanoma on his left leg, which spread to the nodes in his groin. His left inguinal nodes were removed, and as a result, he experiences swelling and discomfort in his leg if he walks or stands for more than an hour. To alleviate the swelling, Paul sits on the floor or a low beach chair and avoids long periods of standing or walking.

Dr. Michael Mastrangelo, an oncologist specializing in melanoma at Thomas Jefferson University Hospital in Philadelphia, says that in his experience, people with groin dissection have a greater problem with swelling than those who undergo dissection in the underarm area. "The side effects of an axillary [underarm] dissection are tolerable. If you were a scratch golfer before, you'll be a scratch golfer after, if you have been rehabilitated." To avoid swelling, doctors recommend the gradual increased use of the arm beginning one to four weeks after the surgery. Swimming, golf, and certain arm exercises are also helpful.

In one study, 25 percent of patients had lymphedema in the legs six months or longer after groin dissection. Only eight percent of these patients suffered significant loss of function of the legs. Swollen legs following groin dissection can be helped by wearing a special supportive stocking and elevating the legs. Below are some suggestions to help keep lymphedema in check:

- Avoid temperature extremes: hot baths, hot tubs, hot showers, Turkish baths, saunas, burns, or travel in extreme climates.
- Avoid infections: insect bites, manicures, pedicures, or other punctures in the affected limb, scratches, cuts.
- Avoid blunt trauma: tight blood pressure cuffs, tight clothing, tight jewelry.

General Precautions
- Maintain a diet low in salt and fatty foods and high in

fresh fruit and vegetables.
- Avoid alcohol and nicotine.
- Avoid excessive weight gain.
- Avoid high-heeled shoes.
- Maintain care of skin and nails.
- Sleep and travel with limbs elevated.
- Swim, walk and participate in other prescribed exercises.
- Use hypoallergenic soap.
- Seek treatment for the slightest lymphedema; treat infections immediately.

Pain, pins-and-needles sensations, and other uncomfortable feelings are common after lymph node dissection. However, for the most part, these problems subside within a few weeks to a few months. In some instances, physical therapy may be necessary to regain strength and range of motion in the affected area.

Undergoing surgery can be disruptive, uncomfortable and frightening. There are always risks associated with surgery, some of them quite serious. Because of this, researchers are very interested in finding out whether elective lymph node dissection increases survival. Experts in this area emphasize that the benefits of elective lymph node dissection versus therapeutic lymph node dissection cannot be resolved based on opinion. The only way to prove that the procedure is worth the risk is to study many patients and observe whether there is a better chance of survival by having the surgery at an early stage. The results of these studies will not be known for at least several more years.

Until then, your physician will be your best source of information and guidance in this area. After carefully analyzing the nature of your primary tumor, your general health, and your personal needs, he or she can help you understand the potential risks and benefits of the procedure.

CHAPTER 10

If Melanoma Returns

A diagnosis of cancer can change a life forever. Even for people whose treatment has proven successful, the possibility of a recurrence—especially of melanoma—is often present. If and when it happens, a recurrence can elicit feelings of hopelessness and despair, a sense that the battle has been lost. Indeed, the statistics associated with recurrence of melanoma can be disheartening. In one study, only 32 percent of patients survived longer than five years after they were diagnosed with a local recurrence (the appearance of tumors near the site of the original melanoma). Recurrences in the lymph nodes and in distant sites of the body significantly decrease the chance for survival. Some people live much longer than average, depending on an array of variables ranging from the size of the tumors, response of the immune system and factors that are still not understood. Also influencing survival is the length of time between original diagnosis and the reappearance of new tumors. A longer "disease-free interval" is associated with longer survival.

The Likelihood of a Recurrence

Recurrence is the appearance of malignant cells from the original tumor in another part of the body some time after the original diagnosis and removal. Your risk for the recurrence of melanoma depends on two factors—the thickness of the primary tumor at the time of its removal and its location on the body.

The thinnest type of melanoma, known as *melanoma in situ*, is considered to be cured with its complete removal. Melanoma in situ is melanoma confined to the epidermis. The National Institutes of Health reported in 1992 that once a melanoma in situ is removed, "there should be no impact on the patient's longevity."

However, every melanoma that is not confined to the epidermis has the potential to recur. The more deeply the melanoma invades, the greater the likelihood of a recurrence. Thicker lesions that have invaded the dermis are sometimes referred to as "high-risk lesions."

Dr. Larry Nathanson of Winthrop University Hospital in Mineola, New York, one of the top melanoma oncologists in the country, has been treating patients for over thirty years. "You must be conservative when reassuring high-risk melanoma patients. Although the first two years after diagnosis remain the period with greatest recurrence rate, we cannot promise patients that they are cured until a very long follow-up time has elapsed."

"Thin non-invasive primary melanoma has a high cure rate; however, it appears that in the small number of patients with thin primaries who do relapse, there is a greater likelihood that they will relapse in more than five years," says Dr. Nathanson.

In the psychological battle against the specter of a recurrence, time is your greatest ally. According to Dr. Alan Houghton of Memorial Sloan-Kettering, "The risk decreases over time, but the highest risk is in the first three years. By three years, the majority of your risk is gone. We have a three-year party, a five-year party and the grand eight-year party. We don't mention cure, but there comes a point where you have to sort it out. I can never tell anybody that they are 100 percent cured of melanoma, but you might be 99 percent cured," he says.

Sites of Recurrence and Associated Therapies

Recurrences can be treated, sometimes quite effectively. It is very important for you to seek medical attention as early as possible if you suspect that your melanoma has returned.

Local Recurrence

Local recurrence is the reappearance of melanoma within approximately five centimeters (about two inches) of the scar of a previously excised melanoma. Unfortunately, a local recurrence may be the signs of malignant cells circulating throughout the body. Most local recurrences develop within five years after the primary melanoma has been removed.

Treatment for a local recurrence varies, depending upon the number of recurrent tumors and other factors. In some cases, the recurrent tumor is surgically removed. This is usually the preferred choice if the original melanoma was thin and there is only one recurrent tumor. In other situations, local recurrence may be treated with isolated limb perfusion (described below), systemic chemotherapy, radiation therapy, injections of immune stimulants, or a combination of these treatments.

In-Transit Recurrent Tumors

In-transit recurrent tumors are growths that appear between the site of the original tumor and the closest lymph node or group of nodes. These tumors appear as small black pebbles or marbles under the skin. They probably originate from tumors traveling within the lymphatic system. Doctors use surgery, systemic chemotherapy, radiation, isolated limb perfusion, immunotherapy or combinations of these to treat in-transit recurrent tumors.

Regional Recurrence

The spread of malignant cells from a primary melanoma to the closest group of lymph nodes form what is known as a *regional recurrence*. These malignant cells can appear in the underarm, groin, neck, or other lymph node areas. Treatment for regional recurrence is limited to lymph node dissection which is discussed in Chapter 9.

Isolated Limb Perfusion

If melanoma reappears on the same arm or leg where it originally occurred, your treatment may include *isolated limb perfusion*. Although isolated limb perfusion has been used to treat several different kinds of cancer, it is most widely and successfully used for the treatment of melanoma. This procedure calls for the delivery of chemotherapy, and more recently, immunologic drugs, only to the limb where the tumors have reappeared. Because only one arm or leg is exposed to these drugs, they can be given in higher doses than could normally be tolerated if administered to the whole body.

Isolated limb perfusion can cause some tumors to disappear and others to shrink so they can be removed more easily with surgery. For individuals who have had a primary melanoma removed from an arm or leg, isolated limb profusion is also being used on an *experimental* basis to determine whether it will delay or prevent tumors from recurring in that limb.

In isolated limb perfusion, circulation to and from the limb is temporarily stopped with a tourniquet. Blood is withdrawn from the limb and pumped through a machine that adds oxygen and anti-cancer drugs. The drugs and limb may be heated to increase the cancer-killing action of the drugs. The blood is then pumped back into the limb.

Isolated limb perfusion is usually accomplished in one treatment, as opposed to a standard course of chemotherapy that may require several visits.

Isolated limb perfusion has not been shown to increase survival on a consistent basis. One study, however, has shown that isolated limb perfusion offers a 20 to 25 percent increase in survival as compared to other types of treatment. Results from several studies indicate that isolated limb perfusion can reduce the size and appearance of tumors in the local area for extended periods of time.

Isolated limb perfusion carries some risks. Almost all patients undergoing isolated limb perfusion experience temporary swelling of the arm or leg. There is also a high risk of bleeding. Blood clots have occurred in 15 percent of patients following isolated limb perfusion. Five percent of patients who undergo this procedure have a temporary reduction in red, white and clotting blood cells. Severe swelling to the arm or leg can occur, and in a very limited number of cases, require amputation.

A similar technique called *intra-arterial regional infusion* is being studied in patients whose disease is limited to the arm or leg. In this procedure, anti-cancer drugs are infused directly into the main artery of the limb, rather than being combined with blood and oxygen.

Living With the Possibility of a Recurrence

"Even though many people who have had cancer are 'doing well,' and might be 'cured,' they often have a lot of psychological distress worrying about a recurrence. In the past, this problem was never attended to, because these people were 'cured.' Only those people who weren't cured medically got our attention," says Dr. Jon Levenson, assistant clinical professor of psychiatry at Columbia-Presbyterian Medical Center in New York. Dr. Levenson is an expert in treating the emotional problems of people with serious illness.

As the number of melanoma and other cancer survivors grows, more consideration is being given to the often difficult psychological effects of living with the possibility of a recurrence. Today, Dr. Levenson and other doctors understand that patients have different ways of dealing with the threat of a recurrence. Some cope with the possibility by healthy denial, meaning that they simply avoid thinking about the disease returning, and do not dwell on it every day. Although denial can be a good way of dealing with the threat of a disease, it can become problematic when it translates into missing doctor's appointments or ignoring symptoms associated with a recurrence, for example. Other patients, of course, have never been in denial and in fact are always mindful of their disease. For them, the concern is that they may dwell upon their condition so frequently that it will interfere with their daily activities. The fine balance between denial and worry is difficult to achieve. In truth, there is no way to know for sure whether cancer will return. It is this uncertainty that changes the life of a person with cancer. The two stories that follow illustrate that sometimes that change can be for the better.

Remembering a Brother

For Senator Connie Mack of Florida, the possibility of a recurrence of melanoma is laden with a painful personal memory. He was already aware of the devastating nature of the disease when he was diagnosed with melanoma in 1989. Just a few years earlier, Senator Mack had been at his younger brother Michael's bedside when he died following a ten-year battle with the disease. Senator Mack admitted that he was very depressed for several years after Michael's death. However, the loss forced him to reassess his own life and motivated him to enter politics. "While Michael's death was the most traumatic experience, it literally changed my life. I asked myself, what's my role, what should I be doing? By forcing myself to deal with those questions, I identified my personal motivation. I wanted to help other people. If it hadn't been for Michael's death, I would have never entered politics."

Years of hard work resulted in the Senator's election to Congress. It was at that time he, too, was diagnosed with melanoma. "Just two months after being sworn into the Senate, I found myself thinking, 'My God, I am going to die.' I went through an instant replay of my brother's death and all of what he went through. I thought, 'Is this the first warning?'" The Senator's melanoma was caught early and he has no signs of advanced disease, but he is left with thoughts that are common for people in his circumstances.

"I still have situations where I get little twinges in the scar where the melanoma was removed and I wonder, 'Is the cancer back?' " Reassured by his doctor that the sensation in his scar was not a cause for concern, Senator Mack has moved ahead and is busy with the responsibilities of his office. The Senator is now working to have a bill passed which will provide a tax credit for individuals who receive early detection tests for certain types of cancer.

Many people, like Senator Mack, are shocked and overwhelmed with anxiety when they are first diagnosed. Gradually, they are able to assess their situation, and find themselves changed. Leslie, an architect in Van Nuys, California, saw a dermatologist in 1979 about a mole on her back. The mole was shaved off and was not considered to be malignant. The mole grew back and, in 1984, Leslie had it biopsied again. This time she was told she had a .07 millimeter melanoma. Instantly, a number of questions raced through her mind. Had the mole been previously misdiagnosed? If so, had it been growing for five years? Was this a recurrence or a new melanoma? She had two children and a husband—what was their future, and hers?

After undergoing a careful evaluation at a university medical center for signs of further spreading, Leslie was told she was free of the disease as far as the doctors could tell. Still, the possibility of a recurrence is now part of her life. "It isn't back now, but I don't want to put it out of my mind. It's like a snake in the grass. You've got to think about it, you've got to watch it. It could return. And I keep telling myself that nobody's safe from everything." Leslie acknowledges that in many ways, having been faced with a serious disease has changed her life in a positive way. "Now when opportunities are within my sight, I go for them. It's like somebody has given me a jewel. My experience with melanoma forced me to take stock of where I was going. I only wish I could have learned this without having the melanoma." A former schoolteacher, Leslie now hopes to work with the American Cancer Society educating children about sun exposure and early melanoma detection.

To date, neither Senator Mack nor Leslie has experienced a recurrence, but both have learned to cope with the possibility that the cancer could return. In doing so, their lives have become more defined. The paradox of cancer affirming life for some has been described by one writer at the National Cancer Institute: "Cancer may rob you of that blissful ignorance that once led you to believe that tomorrow stretched forever. In exchange, you are granted the vision to see each day as precious, a gift to be used wisely and richly. No one can take that away."

CHAPTER 11

Traditional Treatments for Advanced Melanoma

In Chapter 10, the spread of melanoma to nearby parts of the body was discussed. *Distant metastasis* is the spread of tumors to parts of the body further away from the primary melanoma. *Distant recurrence* of melanoma is the reappearance of tumors at distant parts of the body after some time has elapsed from the original diagnosis.

The two most common parts of the body where melanoma cells spread and form distant tumors are the skin and non-regional lymph nodes. Other common areas are the lungs, liver, brain, and bone. However, melanoma can spread to almost any part of the body. Regardless of where it spreads, it is still considered to be melanoma. For instance, if melanoma spreads to the lung, it is still considered to be melanoma and not lung cancer. Doctors are able to determine that tumors appearing in other parts of the body are from the primary melanoma based on microscopic evaluations of the distant tumors.

A careful physical examination is the most effective way to screen for melanoma that might have spread. In addition, a blood test may detect early signs of cancer in the body. A chest X-ray is also routinely given. Generally, a bone, brain and liver scan are not done unless symptoms are present that suggest tumors may be in those areas.

If you are at risk for the spread of melanoma, some of the symptoms that should be brought to your doctor's attention include: weight loss, headache, persistent bone pain, and lumps in the skin.

Treatment for distant recurrence or metastasis may include surgery, radiation, chemotherapy, or experimental therapies such as immunotherapy. Unfortunately, none of these treatments has proven to be effective in curing melanoma. While some people obtain benefits from these therapies, and a very small percentage are even cured, there is no "magic bullet" once the melanoma has spread.

"The paradox of melanoma is that it is a highly curable disease when it is treated early. On the other hand, when it is metastatic it is relatively resistant to treatment by drugs or radiation. With these treatments and even newer types of treatments, we are talking about increases of survival in months," says oncologist Dr. Larry Nathanson.

Only two to three percent of patients with distant melanoma metastasis survive five years. There can be variability in survival depending on the number and location of tumors. Sometimes metastatic tumors grow rapidly, but in other cases they can remain unchanged for extended periods.

How Melanoma Spreads

Metastatic cancer, melanoma included, is made up of many cells that are different from one another. One type of treatment may be effective for killing some types of cells, but others persist and multiply unaffected.

All of the cells that are in a metastatic tumor were originally derived from the cells of the primary tumor. A primary melanoma tumor is made up of cells that are biologically diverse, meaning different from each other in their rate of growth and aggressiveness. Some malignant cells from a primary tumor have the ability to spread to, and grow in, distant sites of the body. Other cells within the same tumor lack the ability to spread.

Dr. Alan Houghton of Memorial Sloan-Kettering explains: "The biology of the tumor is such that whether or not you are going to develop metastases has to do with the original tumor itself and its characteristics. Most of the chain of events that lead up to whether or not it will metastasize may have already occurred by the time the lesion is diagnosed."

The sequence of events leading to metastasis can be explained in this way: As the primary tumor grows, it penetrates more deeply into the layers of the skin. New blood vessels develop to feed the tumor. A cell or group of cells breaks off from the primary tumor and enters the bloodstream or lymphatic system. While traveling through the circulatory system, these cells stick to the walls of blood vessels and penetrate them to enter specific organs. Malignant cells that enter the lymphatic system can travel to the lymph nodes or other organs as well. In order to multiply and develop into metastases, malignant cells must have a supply of oxygen and nutrients. To do this, they induce the growth of new blood vessels. While satisfying their needs, cancer cells destroy healthy cells and tissue.

The presence of tumor cells circulating within the blood vessels, however, does not always mean that metastasis will occur. Less than one percent of melanoma cells injected into laboratory animals were viable 24 hours later and less than 0.1 percent produced metastases, according to experiments completed by Isaiah J. Fidler, Chairman of the Department of Cell Biology at the M.D. Anderson Cancer Center in Houston. What happens to the malignant cells that do not survive? Most of these cells are destroyed by collisions with other cells and vessel walls during their transport in the bloodstream. Our own immune defenses are probably responsible for the destruction of others.

Among other factors, the number of melanoma tumor cells that are released into the bloodstream is related to the thickness of the original melanoma and how long it has been present.

Sorting Out the Explanations

In 1889, London surgeon Stephen Paget posed a question that has puzzled cancer researchers to this day. "What is it that decides what organs shall suffer in a case of disseminated cancer?" In attempting to answer his own query, Dr. Paget suggested that the spread of cancer was due to the fact that certain tumor cells ("the seed") have a specific affinity for certain organs ("the soil"). After more than a century of scientific scrutiny, Dr. Paget's theory still has considerable support.

Modern scientific discoveries have expanded on the seed and soil theory. The ability of malignant cells to invade the surrounding tissues of particular organs seems to be related to complex chemical reactions between the circulating cancer cells and the target organ. Scientists now think that the organ itself produces particular chemicals that support the growth of a tumor. Specialized "seed" cells do not grow randomly in any organ, but only in the "soil" of the target organ that supports its growth.

In experiments with mice, melanoma cells with a tendency to metastasize to the lung were identified and cultivated in a laboratory. Healthy lung tissue was then implanted into the thigh of a mouse. When injected into these mice, the specifically-developed melanoma cells spread selectively to the implanted lung tissue even though it was in the animal's thigh.

Another theory suggests that the spread of cancer depends solely on the number of malignant cells that are sent to an organ and the distance between it and the original tumor. According to this theory, cancer cells that break off from the primary tumor are more likely to metastasize in the closest organ in which the malignant cells are trapped.

The latest theories about the spread of cancer suggest that oncogenes (genes that cause cancer) may play a role in metastasis. Doctors have identified a set of genes (tumor suppressor genes) that are absent in aggressive metastatic melanoma tumors. They theorize that the loss of this gene might contribute to a melanoma cell's potential for metastasis. They have also found that patients with high levels of this gene did somewhat better than patients with low levels. This research suggests that someday metastasis may be controlled by injecting anti-metastatic genes into aggressive tumors to alter their behavior.

As we learn more about metastasis, it appears that no single theory explains the process completely, yet they all provide us with clues that may eventually help solve this puzzle.

The Growth Rate of Cancer Cells

Unregulated growth is one of the hallmarks of malignant cells.

Because most experts agree that a metastatic tumor starts with an individual malignant cell, destruction of 99.9 percent of the malignant cells may still leave enough of them behind to proliferate. Total cure, therefore, may only be achieved if one hundred percent of the cells are destroyed. This fact makes treating metastatic cancer extremely difficult.

Malignant cells can develop an increased ability to invade and spread. This is known as tumor progression. As new malignant cells acquire a greater capacity to invade, spread, and grow rapidly, they become more difficult to kill. Malignant cells have genetic instabilities within them, and, in more advanced cancer, a higher rate of mutation, which produce biologically diverse cells. The changing nature of cancer cells limits the effectiveness of many types of cancer treatments.

Traditional Treatment for Metastatic Melanoma
Surgery

From ancient times to the present, surgery to remove malignant tumors has been employed to cure cancer. As described earlier, the removal of a primary melanoma is usually a simple procedure, requiring only local anesthesia. Surgery to remove tumors that have spread to other parts of the body, however, usually requires general anesthesia and hospitalization. All surgery carries small but significant risks of infection, bleeding, and other problems.

For a small number of patients with advanced stages of the disease, surgery may prolong survival. "There are patients who were found to have a single metastatic site after a careful staging work-up in whom there is no question that surgery seems to be a benefit. Unfortunately, 75 percent of patients with advanced disease have multiple metastatic tumor sites and surgery will probably not benefit this group," says Dr. Larry Nathanson.

Surgery can also help to reduce pain and other symptoms associated with the disease. For example, a metastatic tumor in the brain can sometimes cause dizziness, headaches, and memory loss. If this tumor is safely removed, many of these symptoms can be controlled.

Radiation

Radiation is the use of high-energy X-rays that inhibit the ability of cells to grow and divide. While it has proven effective in the treatment of other kinds of cancer, radiation's application for the treatment of metastatic melanoma is now limited to the relief of symptoms, rather than an increased survival rate or a cure.

For patients with metastatic melanoma, radiation can be used to relieve pain and reduce swelling associated with the presence of a tumor. It is particularly useful in relieving discomfort caused by tumors that occur in the spine.

Several recent experimental treatments combine radiation with heat. Other types of specialized radiation are being tested on melanoma that has spread to the brain. These innovative therapies are promising, but today radiation's major role in metastatic melanoma is to alleviate discomfort when surgery is not a practical alternative.

Chemotherapy

Chemotherapy, the treatment of disease with chemicals or drugs, was discovered in 1910 and was initially used to fight syphilis and other infectious diseases. Its current and primary use as a cancer-killing agent began over 30 years later when, in December, 1943, a United States naval vessel sank in an Italian harbor and its cargo of mustard gas exploded. A number of sailors aboard died from exposure to this poisonous substance. Autopsies revealed that the gas had inhibited the reproduction of white blood cells in the sailors' bodies. This finding led scientists to speculate that the chemicals in mustard gas might help fight leukemia and cancers of the lymphatic system by inhibiting the growth of malignant white blood cells. Experiments with laboratory animals proved the theory, and the age of chemotherapy for the treatment of cancer began.

Since 1955 over 700,000 compounds have been tested for anti-cancer properties. Today the term chemotherapy includes drugs which poison cancer cells (cytotoxic drugs), hormonal agents and a broad spectrum of immunologic drugs that work with the immune system to kill cancer cells.

Treating Cancer with Chemotherapy

As the history of its discovery shows, chemotherapy can be toxic. With chemotherapy, there is a fine line between killing cancer cells and damaging normal ones.

Cancer cells and normal cells are similar in many ways, making the task of destroying cancer cells without harming healthy ones particularly daunting. Chemotherapy may effectively kill all the cancer cells in a person's body, but it can also cause permanent damage to healthy organs.

One of the major differences between cancer cells and healthy cells is their rate of division. Cancer cells proliferate more rapidly than their normal counterparts. Most chemotherapeutic drugs are designed to identify and destroy rapidly proliferating cells. Several types of normal cells, such as cells in the digestive tract, blood cells forming in the bone marrow, and hair follicles proliferate rapidly. Unfortunately, chemotherapeutic drugs can damage these normal cells as the drug circulates through the body.

Moreover, killing all the proliferating cells may not be enough. A sub-group of resting or non-proliferating malignant cells can escape destruction. This phenomenon is called *kinetic resistance*. One way to overcome kinetic resistance is to stimulate these resting cells into a proliferating state. Certain types of chemotherapeutic drugs have been designed to turn resting cells into active ones, but it is unclear what contribution toward cure is made by these drugs.

In order for a chemotherapeutic drug to be effective, it must be able to reach the cancer cells and the cancer cells must be affected by the drug.

The resistance of some cancer cells to a cytotoxic drug is an inherent property of the cancer cell itself and is considered to be permanent. Temporary resistance to a chemotherapeutic drug occurs when the drug cannot reach the cancer cells. For example, tumors in the central nervous system (the brain and spinal cord) are separated from general circulation by the blood-brain barrier, making it difficult for chemotherapeutic drugs to reach these areas.

Treating cancer is also made difficult by the fact that some malignant cells may develop an acquired drug resistance. This means that cells and their progeny may change over time and acquire resistance to a particular drug. As they change, they may develop the ability to survive chemotherapeutic drugs.

Despite these problems, many researchers believe that there are good reasons to continue working with chemotherapy. Certain types of cancer such as Hodgkin's Disease can be cured with the use of chemotherapy and radiation. Chemotherapy can also alleviate pain and other symptoms associated with malignancy.

Chemotherapeutic drugs for melanoma are mainly used for the treatment of advanced disease. At present, there is no consistent evidence that chemotherapy delays or prevents melanoma from recurring after it has been surgically removed.

Chemotherapy for Advanced Melanoma
Single-Agent Chemotherapy

The most commonly used drug for metastatic melanoma is Dacarbazine (DTIC). About 15 to 20 percent of metastatic melanoma tumors respond to this drug, meaning that the tumors show some signs of shrinkage. Unfortunately, these tumors often begin to grow again after a few months. According to Dr. Houghton, about five percent of patients have a complete "clinical response" to DTIC. A complete clinical response is the disappearance of all detectable tumor based on tests such as X-rays and nuclear scans. Undetectable amounts of cancer cells can still be present in the body. These undetectable growths called *micrometastases* can multiply and become apparent in the body at a later point.

People undergoing treatment with DTIC can usually continue with the normal activities of their life. Unlike other types of chemotherapy, DTIC does not cause hair loss or affect a person's blood count, according to Dr. Houghton. The most common side effect of DTIC is nausea and vomiting, usually worse on the first day of treatment. Some people may experience diarrhea, fatigue, and flu-like symptoms. DTIC may be administered on varying schedules—a one-day treatment repeated at three-week intervals, a five-day treatment every three weeks, or a ten-day treatment repeated every four weeks. DTIC is usually administered into the vein and can be completed on an out-patient basis in most cases.

"DTIC is a very reasonable option if you balance it against everything else," Dr. Houghton says. "Any patient should understand that response to chemotherapy or any treatment does not mean cure, it means shrinkage of a tumor, usually most of it, but not disappearance. With DTIC, the response lasts four to eight months on the average. But that means that half of the people who took it had a response time that was less than that, and the other half had more. So there may be a group of patients whose response can last years."

To date, DTIC is the only drug approved by the FDA for the treatment of melanoma, but doctors use other types of chemotherapy as well. A drug not yet available for use in the United States is Fotemustine. In preliminary studies, the response rate for Fotemustine has been somewhat higher than the response for DTIC. In addition, Fotemustine appears to have some effect on melanoma that has spread to the brain and the central nervous system, areas that most chemotherapeutic drugs cannot reach because of the blood-brain barrier.

Taxol, a new drug originally derived from the bark of the western yew tree, has been shown to have some value in fighting melanoma based on laboratory studies.

Combination Chemotherapy

Because of the relatively poor results of single-agent chemotherapy, researchers have tried to improve response rates by using combinations of various drugs. In theory, the advantage of combination drug therapy is that several drugs can be given at once or in close proximity to each other and increase the possibility that cancer cells will be killed in different ways. These combinations have more side effects than DTIC alone. Patients should understand, however, that long-term increases in survival rates for advanced melanoma, even with combinations of these drugs, have not yet been achieved on a consistent basis.

One of the more promising combinations of drugs is the Dartmouth Regime, developed at the Dartmouth Medical Center in 1984. This therapy consists of DTIC, cisplatin and BCNU (chemotherapeutic drugs), and tamoxifen (a hormone-blocking compound). Patients undergoing this regime will usually require a hospital stay of three to four days. It is not known whether the Dartmouth Regime is more effective than DTIC alone because studies comparing the two treatments have not been completed.

Dr. Nathanson recently completed a study using the three chemotherapeutic drugs from the Dartmouth Regime, but substituting a different hormonal agent called megestrol acetate (Megase) for tamoxifen. This hormonal agent has been shown to prevent loss of appetite and loss of weight, a common and serious problem in cancer patients undergoing chemotherapy. According to Dr. Nathanson, megestrol acetate does not have a direct anti-tumor effect against melanoma, but augments the anti-tumor properties of the chemotherapeutic drugs with which it is combined. His data showed that patients using this regime had increased survival rates compared to the Dartmouth Regime.

There are many other combination chemotherapy regimes now being tested. Each combination has varying side effects and potential benefits.

Fighting the Odds

Dr. Michael Mastrangelo is an expert on melanoma and the use of chemotherapy to treat it. He believes that, in some cases, chemotherapy for melanoma patients, although difficult and uncertain, is worth trying.

"I don't think that anybody should die without the opportunity for chemotherapy. When someone takes chemotherapy, he or she is gambling quality of life against a home run. If you treat a group of people with aggressive chemotherapy, there is the prospect that someone in the group can have the disease go into complete remission and, I believe, a prospect for a cure. Other doctors may just tell melanoma patients to get their affairs in order, but I approach every case as if I am going to win. Almost invariably, I portray hope, because I have seen people snatched from the jaws of death, and I assume that the next person I see will be that person. If I am treating you, you are never without treatment. You are never without someone telling you that you are going to make it."

Dr. Mastrangelo believes that there is reason for cautious optimism about the usefulness of chemotherapy for melanoma. Yet other researchers feel that since the chance of chemotherapy affecting long-term survival is poor, patients with advanced melanoma should consider entering into experimental studies for other new treatments. This difficult decision should be made after a complete discussion with your doctor and others whose advice you value.

Besides single-agent and combination chemotherapy, researchers are studying the effectiveness of chemotherapy used with immunotherapy. This approach combines the cancer-killing effect of chemotherapy with immune-bolstering substances.

Choosing Treatment
Weighing the Factors

In her comprehensive book *Coping with Chemotherapy*, Nancy Bruning, a nurse and cancer patient, writes: "The decision to undergo chemotherapy cannot be made . . . unless you have gathered enough pertinent information to allow you to assess the risks versus the benefits for you, in your particular circumstances. Your doctor is your primary source of information and advice. But it should not be left up to him to make the final decision—or to provide all the information you might need in order to make the choice."

Making a treatment choice for chemotherapy requires a careful balancing of priorities and a clear understanding of your goals.

"It's a patient's choice," says Dr. Houghton. "Do you want the most aggressive therapy where your chances might be better, or a better quality of life from day to day? Some patients want me to decide for them, so I try to find out whether they wish to continue working every day and enjoying their general good health, or whether they want to take a risk, knowing that our data is limited, that the drugs we use may cause them to feel ill but may benefit them in the long-run."

By discussing potential side effects and risks with your doctor before undergoing treatment, you will gain the perspective and understanding that will help you make the choice that is best for you.

Side Effects of Chemotherapy

The prospect of undergoing chemotherapy causes many patients to worry. Some have a vague but real fear of chemotherapy, usually from what they have heard or from seeing a family member or a friend go through it. Keep in mind that great advances have been made in alleviating the side effects of chemotherapy. For example, new drugs can block signals in your brain that can trigger vomiting when chemotherapy is administered. Many of these drugs have been developed only in the last 15 years.

Mary Patricia McGovern, an oncology nurse at Columbia-Presbyterian Medical Center in New York, says that improving the chemotherapy experience can be achieved through effective communication between doctor, patient and chemotherapy nurse. "Feelings of fear about chemotherapy need to be validated. Patients need to know that they are allowed to be afraid. Beyond that, patients need to know what to expect."

Ms. McGovern candidly admits that it is often the oncology nurse rather than the oncologist who is the source for emotional and educational support when it comes to chemotherapy.

Nausea and Vomiting

Certain types of drugs used to treat melanoma, including DTIC, cisplatin, BCNU, and CCNU, among others, cause nausea and vomiting. Anti-nausea drugs can be administered directly into a vein along with or after the administration of chemotherapy. Commonly used anti-nausea drugs include the following:

Prochlorperazine (Compazine): In use for 20 years, it is available in many forms, including pill, rectal suppository or injection. Side effects include drowsiness, low blood pressure and jitteriness.

Metoclopramide (Reglan): This drug can be helpful in preventing nausea with even the most nauseating chemotherapy drugs. Side effects include drowsiness, diarrhea, restlessness and anxiety.

Ondansetron (Zofran): A relatively new anti-nausea drug that is now available in tablet form, it is very effective for alleviating nausea associated with DTIC. Ondanestron doesn't have the side effects of other types of anti-nausea drugs. The most common side effect is headache or constipation.

Besides anti-nausea medications, there are certain things that you can do to lessen stomach upset. The National Cancer Institute recommends the following:

- Avoid big meals. Eat several small meals throughout the day.
- Drink liquids at least an hour before or after mealtime, instead of with your meals.
- Eat and drink slowly.
- Eat foods cold or at room temperature so you won't be bothered by strong smells.
- Drink cool, clear, unsweetened fruit juices, such as apple

or grape juice, or light-colored sodas, such as ginger ale, which have lost their fizz.

- Try to avoid odors that bother you, such as cooking smells, smoke or perfume.
- Breathe deeply and slowly when you feel nauseated.
- Avoid eating for at least a few hours before treatment if nausea usually occurs during chemotherapy.

Hair Loss
DTIC usually does not cause hair loss, but another type of chemotherapy drug used to treat melanoma, vincristine and certain other drugs can do so.

Usually, hair will grow back normally after you have completed your course of chemotherapy. If you notice some hair loss, remember to use mild shampoos, soft-bristled hair brushes, and avoid rollers, dyes and permanents.

If you choose to cover your head, here are a few tips:

- Get your wig or hairpiece before you lose a lot of hair so you can match your natural color and style. (On the other hand, one woman who lost her hair during chemotherapy for melanoma decided to try a wig that was a different color from her own hair. She thought that the color was so flattering that she dyed her hair that shade when it grew back.)
- Consider borrowing a wig or hairpiece rather than purchasing one. Check with the local chapter of the American Cancer Society or with the social work department of your hospital. You might also choose to buy scarves, turbans or hats that look attractive and may be more comfortable than a wig.
- A hairpiece that is needed because of cancer treatment is tax-deductible and might be covered by your health insurance.

Other Side Effects

Some chemotherapeutic drugs can adversely affect the growth of cells in your bone marrow, predisposing you to anemia, infection and bleeding.

Anemia is a low red blood cell count which may cause you to feel tired. Your doctor will monitor you for this condition. If your red blood cell count is too low, you may need a blood transfusion to increase the number of red blood cells in your body. During these difficult times, remember to ask for help if you need it from family and friends. It is important that you rest when you feel tired.

Chemotherapy may also decrease the ability of your bone marrow to produce white blood cells. As a result, you may become susceptible to infection. Check with your doctor when and if this condition is most likely to occur. To avoid infections, here are some suggestions:

- Wash your hands often during the day, especially after using the bathroom.
- Stay away from people who have diseases you might catch, such as a cold, flu, measles or chicken pox.
- Don't cut or tear the cuticles of your nails.
- Be careful not to nick or cut yourself.
- Use an electric shaver instead of a razor.
- Use a soft toothbrush that won't hurt your gums.
- Don't squeeze or scratch pimples.
- Take a warm (not hot) bath, shower or sponge bath every day. Pat your skin dry using a light touch—don't rub.

Signs of an infection should be brought to the attention of your doctor immediately. They include: fever over 100 degrees Fahrenheit; chills; sweating; loose bowels (this can also be a side effect of chemotherapy); a burning sensation when you urinate; a cough or sore throat; unusual vaginal discharge or itching; any redness or swelling, especially around a wound, sore, pimple, or boil.

Don't use any aspirin or other medicine to bring your temperature down without first checking with your doctor.

Another side effect of chemotherapy is blood clotting problems. Platelets, reduced by chemotherapy, are cells that are important in helping blood clot. If your blood does not have enough platelets, you may bleed or bruise more easily. Let your doctor know if you notice unexpected bruising, small red spots under the skin, pink or red colored urine or black or bloody stool. You may also notice small amounts of bleeding from your gums or nose. If your platelet count falls too low, you may need a platelet transfusion

There are many books and pamphlets that your doctor can provide which have information about appropriate food choices and cooking that will help you feel better during chemotherapy. (See Appendix for list of recommended books.)

Ask your doctor or chemotherapy nurse to help you contact community organizations or the American Cancer Society, a visiting nurse association, or other social welfare services that can assist you during chemotherapy.

Choosing Where to Receive Treatment

Chemotherapy for melanoma is usually introduced into the body with a needle inserted into a vein in the hand or arm. The liquid flows from a container into the body. Generally, this takes place in a doctor's office or a hospital clinic. Sometimes a patient may remain in the hospital for observation, but in most cases, he or she can go home.

The question of where a patient should go for chemotherapy treatment needs to be addressed by both the patient and family members. Some people prefer treatment to be close to home, or at a site that is accessible by public transportation. Others will travel great distances to facilities that have national reputations for cancer care. Some may be interested in entering into experimental trials of new drug therapies available only at certain facilities.

There are 57 Cancer Treatment Centers in the United States (see Appendix). Forty of them are specifically devoted to the diagnosis and treatment of cancer patients, and most have additional support facilities for rehabilitation and follow-up care. Out of those 40, 24 are Comprehensive Cancer Treatment Centers which meet the criteria of the National Cancer Institute. If you do not live near a Comprehensive Cancer Treatment Center, it may be worthwhile to discuss with your doctor the possibility of referral to one for evaluation. Often, your doctor can care for you at a community hospital or other local facility after an initial evaluation at a Cancer Center. This option may allow you to be near your personal physician and family but still have the benefit of the most up-to-date information provided by the center.

Nancy Bruning advises: "If you are a patient who has an unusual or difficult cancer and for whom the standard or the local investigational treatment leaves much to be desired, it may definitely be worthwhile for you to travel to see highly experienced specialists. Another valid reason for seeking treatment at a cancer center is when it is the only source for a particular experimental program that might help you."

Convenience and comfort are vital, so before deciding on a treatment center you should tour the facility. Look to see if there is adequate privacy, pleasant surroundings, and insulation from noise and traffic. If you choose a facility that is far from home, check with the social services department to find out if there are hotels or other living quarters in the area where your family can stay while you are being treated.

Chemotherapy nurses are specially trained in both the physical and the emotional aspects of cancer. They will be an important part of your care and their attitude can greatly affect your experience. Try to meet with the chemotherapy nurses at the facility you are considering. Do they seem caring, unhurried, professional, easy to talk to? The answers to these questions should influence your decision on where to receive your treatment.

The atmosphere of the facility where you receive chemotherapy can have a significant impact on how you feel. Glenn, whose battle with melanoma included chemotherapy, had two very different experiences with his treatment that were related not to new drugs or increased dosages but to the environment of the facility. At one hospital, "everything went wrong," according to Glenn. "It was gloomy. When they gave you the chemo, they would just leave you there. When the bag [of chemotherapy] was empty, you had to wait for someone to come by to change it." The ambiance at this facility affected him physically, and for the first time in the course of his treatment, he vomited.

In contrast, Glenn says that the facility to which he switched was cheerier and friendlier. "The nurses sit you down in a recliner, and they take care of everything. They give you something to relax, and are right there to change the bag when it runs out." Although these differences may seem minor, they had a very real impact on him.

The idea of receiving chemotherapy can be very stressful for patients. It is a good idea to plan ahead and make informed decisions about the facility where you will be treated to avoid anxiety or stress.

Refusing Chemotherapy or Any Treatment

For some people, the decision to try chemotherapy to over-come melanoma may be filled with concern and apprehension. Drugs now available for the treatment of melanoma show only limited responses. Some patients choose not to try chemotherapy or any treatment because they believe that the side effects will interfere with the quality of their lives. Others choose experimental therapies in the hope that the newer types of treatment may yield better results or help future patients. Some doctors recommend that certain patients try experimental therapies, such as vaccines and other biological modifiers, before trying chemotherapy. This is because chemotherapy may weaken your immune system, making immunotherapy less effective. You should discuss this option with your doctor to see if you are a candidate for these or other therapies.

Ultimately, forgoing treatment after considering all other options might be the right choice for certain people. It is a highly personal decision that only you can make.

$\langle \rangle$

CHAPTER 12

Experimental Treatments for Advanced Melanoma

Chemotherapy, surgery, and radiation, the cornerstones of cancer treatment, have been only modestly successful in combating advanced melanoma. Yet some scientists still believe we can cure melanoma with existing therapies by utilizing them more efficiently. Others advocate new and innovative approaches such as cancer vaccines, which stimulate and enhance our immune system. Still other scientists think that combining traditional and experimental therapies is the answer.

For a patient confronted with advanced melanoma, the decision to forgo traditional treatment, in favor of investigational methods, may seem like a reasonable alternative. Some people, however, are frightened by the thought of trying an unproven treatment in the search for an elusive cure they may never enjoy. Of this concern, Nancy Bruning writes: "Participating in an investigational trial gives patients an opportunity to receive state-of-the-art treatment—imperfections and all—that would not otherwise be available and that can make a vast difference in their prognoses."

If a new treatment is successful, those brave patients receiving it will be the first to benefit. There are certain risks, however, that you should consider. Although all treatment studies have built-in safeguards to protect patients, new treatments can produce unanticipated side effects. Furthermore, not all patients in every study receive the new treatment. Some are in a control group that receives standard care for comparison to the new approach.

Therapy that attempts to prevent the recurrence of melanoma after all signs of the cancer have been eliminated (adjuvant therapy) and treating advanced melanoma are the major goals of clinical trials in this field. New combinations of traditional chemotherapy, tumor-targeted radiation and exciting applications of advances in immunology and genetic therapy are some of the specific methods being investigated by scientists today.

Choosing Experimental Therapy

At this time, most melanoma patients who participate in clinical trials have not done better than patients being treated with traditional therapy. However, for many patients, experimental therapy offers intangible psychological advantages. A patient may feel he or she is in greater control of the disease, and life in general, by participating in such therapy. In addition, a small chance to improve life expectancy or decrease symptoms associated with the disease may be worth the effort.

Patients using experimental therapy for advanced disease may have already tried traditional treatments such as surgery and chemotherapy but have had poor results and are willing to try something as yet unproven. Others may decide to try experimental therapy even before undergoing traditional treatment. A person may be treated with both traditional and experimental therapies at the same time. In certain clinical trials, however, a patient may only be accepted into a program if he or she has not used chemotherapy or immunotherapy.

A patient entering into a clinical trial should understand the experimental nature of the treatment. There are no guarantees. Instead, there is the promise that each participant is bringing the prospects for a cure closer.

Trials to Prevent a Recurrence

The best candidates for experimental adjuvant therapy are those who have had surgical removal of lymph nodes containing melanoma but no further evidence of spread to major organs. Other possible candidates are patients who have a relatively thick melanoma (greater than two millimeters in some studies or greater than four in others) without other signs of disease, according to Dr. Alan Houghton. In short, the best candidates for experimental adjuvant therapy are those people who are relatively healthy but are at a high risk for recurrence.

Clinical Trials

If you are considering participating in a clinical trial, your *informed consent* is needed. Informed consent means that you have been apprised of the risks and potential benefits of the trial and are willing to participate. You will receive a printed consent form that should be written in language that is understandable to you. Before signing the form that gives your consent, your physician should review the following information with you:

• A complete description of the intended treatment
• A list of potential side effects and risks
• A discussion of other treatments that may be beneficial

The National Cancer Institute suggests that if you are considering entering a trial, you ask the following questions:

• What is the purpose of the study?
• What does the study involve? What kinds of tests and treatments will I have to undergo?

- What is likely to happen to me with or without this new research treatment?
- What are my other choices? What are their advantages and disadvantages?
- How could this study affect my daily life? (travel time, in- or out-patient procedures)
- What side effects can I expect?
- How long will this study last?
- Will this experimental therapy keep me from getting other types of treatment?

You can choose to discontinue participation in a trial at any point. You should never feel pressured to remain in a trial if you are uncomfortable with any aspect of it or if you simply want to stop participating for no reason at all. Before discontinuing, however, try to speak with your doctor to discuss your concerns.

Phases of Drug Evaluation

The National Cancer Institute coordinates clinical trials using doctors and investigators who oversee the programs on a voluntary basis. On the average, it takes ten to twelve years from the date of its discovery for a new drug to be marketed and approved for use.

After drugs are tested on animals in a laboratory, those that may be useful to humans are subjected to four phases of testing with patients. Generally speaking, a patient only participates in one phase of a trial, depending on his or her health and prior treatments.

Preclinical Phase: The drugs are tested in rodents and then in large animals.

Phase I: This phase is usually offered to patients with advanced stages of a cancer who have tried several types of therapies that have failed. The goal of a Phase I study is to find the best way to administer a new treatment and how much of it can be given safely. The drug dosage is gradually increased in subsequent patients until the dose that produces tolerable side effects is reached. Patients who participate in Phase I trials need to be closely monitored and available at the treatment center to be observed on a regular basis.

Phase II: The anti-tumor activity of the drug is tested. The tumors are measured before and after treatment to determine the amount of drugs needed to produce a response with tolerable side effects.

Phase III: If the drug is found to be beneficial, it is used in Phase III trials and a comparison of its usefulness and side effects versus drugs currently being used takes place with a large group of patients.

Phase IV: The new drug is incorporated into primary treatment in combination with standard drugs.

For specific information about clinical trials in your area, and the costs involved, call the National Cancer Institute's Cancer Information Service at 1-800-4-CANCER.

Our Immune System: A Natural Cancer Killer

Many scientists believe that the cure for melanoma lurks within the complex workings of our own immune system. More than many other cancers, melanoma seems to stimulate the body's natural mechanisms that seek out and destroy malignant cells. It was one of the first human tumors in which scientists actually observed an immune response. Scientists looking at melanomas under the microscope often see cells produced by the immune system attacking the malignancy.

One of the most important components of the immune system are lymphocytes—a type of white blood cell which travels throughout the body and attacks bacteria, viruses, and cancer cells. Lymphocytes are of particular importance in the study of melanoma and the immune system. In fact, extracts of human melanoma tumors have been shown to stimulate lymphocytes. There are two types of lymphocytes. B-lymphoctyes produce antibodies, molecules that attach to foreign proteins signaling other immune cells to attack them. T-lymphocytes can stimulate an immune reaction or kill tumors directly.

The immune system works continually to destroy cancer cells that may be floating in the body and reduces the chance that these malignant cells will multiply and form a tumor mass. However, the immune system can sometimes fail to recognize malignant cells because they often resemble healthy cells. In his book *The Transformed Cell*, Dr. Steven A. Rosenberg, an authority on experimental treatment of melanoma, describes the workings of the immune system this way:

> Just as police use fingerprints to identify a suspect, the immune system reads the markings on cells and chemicals within the body to distinguish between that which does belong, or "self," and that which does not belong, or "non-self." ...But just as fingerprints can be smeared or hard to read, making it difficult to identify a suspect, the self and non-self markings can be obscured, making it difficult for the immune system to identify a target.

The goal of immunotherapy is to improve the way the body detects and fights cancer. Immunotherapy, also known as biological therapy, works in several different ways. It can:

1. Directly kill malignant cells.
2. Change the way the body reacts to a tumor.
3. Suppress body responses that permit cancer growth.
4. Make a cancer cell more sensitive to destruction.

Spontaneous Regression

Host response is a medical term for the reaction by the patient's own immune system to a disease. The "host" refers to the individual who has an unwanted guest—-an infection or cancer. Many experts believe that host response may cause the occasional spontaneous disappearance of melanoma, also known as *spontaneous regression.* Spontaneous regression means the disappearance or shrinkage of cancer cells without medical intervention. This phenomenon rarely occurs, but it does happen more frequently with primary melanoma than almost any other type of cancer. It suggests that our bodies have the capacity to recognize and destroy melanoma cells on their own. The black tumors of melanoma sometimes turn white as they shrink during spontaneous regression. Many scientists believe this is the result of the immune system attacking malignant pigmented cells and destroying them.

Natural antibodies against melanoma have been discovered in the blood of approximately one-third of patients with the disease. This finding suggests that the body, without the aid of any outside therapy, can begin to fight against cancer cells. Antibodies, one of the most active components of the immune system, form a complex surveillance network which identifies and tracks down enemies, such as cancer cells.

Aided by such an impressive array of natural cancer killers, scientists are trying to design therapies which use and amplify our inherent immune mechanisms. Attempts are being made to enhance the body's cancer-fighting potential by using natural substances such as interferon and interleukin-2. In addition, researchers are now using vaccines derived from the melanoma tumor itself in an attempt to halt its spread or return.

Types of Immunotherapy
Non-Specific Immunostimulants

There are several ways to utilize immunotherapy in an attempt to treat melanoma. The earliest and best studied approach is with non-specific immunostimulants. These agents "rev up" the immune system in a general way and may cause the body to attack abnormal cells, such as cancer cells, more aggressively. The goal of non-specific immune therapy is to increase the body's resistance to everything, not just one specific disease. BCG (*Bacillus* Calmette-Guerin), a vaccine that has long been used to immunize patients against tuberculosis, has been studied as a therapy for melanoma. BCG is administered intralesionally, meaning that it is injected directly into a melanoma tumor on the skin. A high proportion of skin lesions have regressed after they were injected with BCG. Despite these promising results, BCG does not appear to be effective in treating melanoma that has spread to major organs, nor does it seem to delay its recurrence.

Specific Immunotherapy: Melanoma Vaccines

The interplay between melanoma and the immune system has led some people to suggest that melanoma may be the first cancer to be defeated by a vaccine. According to Jean-Claude Bystryn, M.D., Professor of Dermatology and Director of the Melanoma Program and Melanoma Immunotherapy Clinic at New York University, spontaneous regression provides strong evidence that the body does have the ability to fight melanoma. Dr. Bystryn has devoted his research to the development and testing of a vaccine that may someday prevent or even cure melanoma. "If you believe that the body has a mechanism to fight cancer—and we have seen cancer go away on its own—then trying to stimulate the immune system is a very reasonable approach. The important principal is that the body can do it and does so routinely. We just have to find ways to make the body do it more effectively," he says.

Although the idea of treating cancer with a vaccine has been considered by scientists for at least a century, the technology needed to produce it has only recently caught up with the underlying theory. Melanoma cells produce numerous proteins called *antigens* which mark the cell as normal or abnormal. When tumor cell antigens are recognized as abnormal, they can trigger an immune response, which usually means that the body sends antibodies and cells to attack the antigens and the cells on which they reside.

In the last several years, the potential effectiveness of the melanoma vaccine has been increased due to the identification of some of these tumor antigens by researchers. By using these specific tumor antigens in a vaccine, the odds of producing an effective immune response may increase.

Dr. Bystryn is working with a vaccine made up of antigens from different human melanoma tumors. The vaccine is polyvalent, meaning that it contains more than one type of antigen. Once they have been concentrated and partly purified in the laboratory, these antigens are then injected into patients. Dr. Bystryn hopes that this will stimulate the immune system to target the patient's own tumors.

While Dr. Bystryn's data shows that patients who develop a strong immune response to vaccines remain cancer-free for longer periods than those patients who have a lesser response, it does not prove that the vaccine will delay a recurrence. In order to prove that a vaccine works, there must be a study which compares patients who use the vaccine with those who do not. These trials are now underway, but the results will not be known for several years. According to Dr. Bystryn, the vaccine has been administered to over 200 patients with very few side effects.

Researchers have tried to improve the immune reaction to vaccines by adding viruses, BCG, and low doses of cyclophosphamide (Cytoxan), a chemotherapy drug. Doctors believe cyclophosphamide enhances the response to vaccines by lowering the activity of cells which suppress immune responsiveness. Certain viruses appear to enhance the immune response as well. Early studies indicate that these substances may improve the level, duration and quality of the immune response to the vaccine.

Dr. Donald Morton, a melanoma specialist now working at the John Wayne Cancer Institute in Santa Monica, has been testing vaccines made from whole melanoma cells grown in the laboratory and then irradiated. His vaccine is composed of three different strains of melanoma cells which contain a high concentration of the six major melanoma-associated antigens. Dr. Morton believes that his new vaccine may have the potential to play an expanded role in the management of melanoma. Further comparative studies are underway which may prove his theories correct.

Case Histories

Some patients with high-risk melanoma (thick primary melanoma) have decided to participate in melanoma vaccine trials after carefully considering their options.

Maureen, a 40-year-old artist from Ohio, had a malignant

melanoma removed from her back in 1987. The disease reappeared in her lymph nodes in 1992. The reappearance of melanoma placed her in a high-risk category and forced her to think about what to do next. Maureen read as much as possible about treatment options and solicited many opinions.

Since Maureen was in good physical shape, relatively young, and willing to travel, she decided to participate in Dr. Bystryn's program. With the help of Corporate Angels Network (an organization that fills available space on corporate-sponsored flights with cancer patients needing transportation to treatment centers) and her family's frequent flyer tickets, Maureen makes the trip to New York to receive her injections. Besides a day or two of flu-like symptoms, she feels well after the treatments and is optimistic that the vaccine was the right choice.

Some patients have had long-term success with vaccines. Sandy Hawley was a champion jockey, winning the Queen's Plate in Montreal and finishing "in the money" at the Kentucky Derby, when his trainer noticed a black mole the size of dime on Sandy's back. The mole was diagnosed as malignant melanoma, and soon thereafter, Sandy underwent an elective lymph node dissection. A single microscopic bit of melanoma was discovered in one node. There was no other traditional treatment available to Sandy, except for regular check-ups. Down but not out, Sandy decided to participate in a vaccine program in California. Since that time, he has had no sign of disease for five years. In addition to the vaccine, Sandy adopted a strict vegetarian diet which he believes helps him maintain good health.

While inspiring, these two stories do not prove that vaccines work. To date, there have been no long-term trials comparing the survival of patients treated with vaccines with patients receiving no treatment. Further research and trials need to be done before the effectiveness of vaccines is known with any certainty.

Other Experimental Therapies
Interferon
Interferon, a naturally-produced protein, has great potential for fighting cancer. It was discovered in 1957, when scientists identified a substance that provided other cells resistance to viral infections. Interferon may work directly by killing tumors, or indirectly by inhibiting tumor growth via the immune system. The problem has always been that interferon is produced in miniscule quantities by the body. For example, scientists who used large amounts of blood products to harvest interferon were only able to extract a final product that was less than two percent pure. By using human tissue as a biological springboard, commercial laboratories were able to produce interferon in greater amounts in the early 1980s. Genetic codes that contain the blueprint to produce interferon were isolated and used as a template by other cells. This is known as recombinant DNA technology. By producing greater quantities of interferon and in a purer form via recombinant DNA techniques, anti-tumor response rates have improved.

One type of interferon, interferon-alpha, has been widely studied and is considered to be a potentially powerful agent for treating metastatic melanoma. Despite this, most patients do not seem to benefit significantly from this drug. Clinical trials with interferon-alpha show that about ten to 20 percent of melanoma patients respond to the treatment and one quarter of the responses are complete remissions. Unfortunately, the responses are generally short-lived. Half of the people who respond to interferon-alpha see their tumors grow again within six months. Higher response rates occurred in patients given interferon-alpha in combination with chemotherapy. In Phase II trials there was a 50 percent reduction in the size of tumors in some patients being treated with this dual therapy. However, many questions about the efficacy of this treatment remain because large-scale studies have not been done.

The side effects of interferon-alpha include flu-like symptoms, muscle soreness, headache, fever, chills, and loss of appetite. Patients should also be aware that interferon-alpha is not F.D.A.-approved for the treatment of melanoma. DTIC is the only F.D.A.-approved drug for melanoma, but many doctors commonly use other drugs on an experimental basis.

Interleukin-2

Interleukin-2 (IL-2) is a molecule produced by lymphocytes that regulates and strengthens the immune response. It has two properties that may help doctors defeat melanoma. First, it can enhance the immune response by stimulating the proliferation of lymphocytes. A lymphocyte that has been exposed to IL-2 and develops the ability to kill cancer cells is called a Lymphokine Activated Killer (LAK) cell. IL-2 and LAK cells have shown heightened anti-tumor activity in animal studies.

Another important use of IL-2 is its ability to induce the growth of Tumor Infiltrating Lymphocytes (TIL). TIL cells are white blood cells that are sometimes found within a melanoma tumor. TIL cells can be isolated from tumors, then treated with IL-2 and re-infused into the patient in an attempt to destroy melanoma cells. Preliminary studies have shown TIL cells to be many times more potent than LAK cells.

Interleukin-2, like interferon, can be produced in a laboratory in greater quantities than are available in the body. In 1982, IL-2 was first seen to activate Natural Killer (NK) cells, lymphocytes that spontaneously kill tumor cells. Partial responses were achieved with high doses of IL-2 in melanoma patients during clinical trials at the National Cancer Institute Surgery Branch. The major obstacle for increasing dosages of IL-2 has been the serious toxic effects this treatment has on patients.

At the National Cancer Institute Surgery Branch in Maryland, Dr. Steven A. Rosenberg has been experimenting with IL-2 and LAK cells for the treatment of several types of cancer, including melanoma. Initial results of his experiments showed a limited number of responses for melanoma, and rare but occasional long-term complete remissions. Other studies of IL-2 have been less encouraging, but research continues.

IL-2 is toxic, especially in high doses. For this reason, candidates for IL-2 trials will not be considered if they have any serious health problems in addition to melanoma. IL-2 is now F.D.A.-approved only for the treatment of metastatic kidney cancer, but physicians are permitted to use it in the management of melanoma. Interleukin-2 is sometimes recommended for patients in good physical condition when more traditional treatments fail.

Monoclonal Antibodies

Discovered in 1975, *monoclonal antibodies* are proteins that can detect tumor cells. They are therefore sometimes "piggybacked" with drugs and radioactive material in an effort to target malignant cells and treat them effectively while sparing healthy cells. Monoclonal antibodies also have properties which allow them to destroy cancer cells on their own. Phase I studies are now in progress around the country to determine the effectiveness of monoclonal antibodies in fighting melanoma.

The Future of Experimental Therapies

As scientists continue to refine the known treatments, others are busy working on entirely new concepts. Dr. Alan Houghton believes that one of the most important pieces of the melanoma puzzle will be found when the gene for malignant melanoma is identified. This discovery would enable doctors to identify persons who are at high risk for the disease and immunize them even before melanoma has a chance to develop.

At Memorial Sloan-Kettering, Dr. Houghton is also exploring the relationship between melanoma and a skin condition called vitiligo in which the immune system attacks normal pigment cells, causing the loss of color. Dr. Houghton explains that melanoma cells resemble normal pigment cells in many ways, much like breast cancer cells resemble normal breast tissue. "A tumor cell is not some aberrant thing, it is not completely different from the normal cells from which it was first derived. A tumor is something that has become uncontrolled, but still retains the characteristics of its normal parent cells," he says.

According to Dr. Houghton, patients who develop vitiligo after being diagonosed with metastatic melanoma have a much better prognosis than patients who do not develop vitiligo. He is now considering the possibility of fighting melanoma with a vaccine directed against normal pigment cells in the hopes that it will produce a reaction against abnormal pigment cells—melanoma—as well.

Another new technique, boron neutron capture therapy (BNCT), may enable doctors to treat melanoma that has spread to the brain, an area that is difficult for chemotherapeutic drugs to reach because of the blood-brain barrier. Scientists send boron to the tumor and then expose the patient a low energy neutron beam. When a neutron beam is captured by the boron atom, there is a release of an enormous amount of energy confined to a very small diameter. Doctors hope they can refine this technique so they can use it to destroy brain tumors.

Faddist or Questionable Remedies

Faced with a progressive and life-threatening disease, and the reality that traditional and even experimental treatments often fail, some patients turn to alternative therapies. One study indicates that followers of alternative medicine are generally upper middle class, well-educated people. Reaching for help outside traditional medicine is an understandable response.

In recent years, holism, homeopathy, herbalism and other non-medical movements have been receiving much attention. In fact, the demand for information about unconventional medical practices has been so great that the National Institutes of Health has recently initiated The Office of Alternative Medicine (O.A.M.). This office is devoted to identifying alternative medicine issues and formulating recommendations related to future research in this area. The work being done at O.A.M. is important because it will provide information about alternative medicine based on scientific and unbiased studies.

To dismiss every non-traditional approach to healing as "mere quackery" does little to discriminate between dangerous unproven methods and helpful approaches that may contribute to a person's well-being. One cancer patient and author writes: "Be as painstaking in checking the credentials of those who offer you holistic services as you would be of other practitioners, whether as leader of a group or as individual therapist. Be wary too of therapists who would deprive you of what modern medicine has to offer you, who will not work with doctors. If therapists are true holists, they will acknowledge the strong powers of the body as well as of the mind and the uncertainties of the complex relationship between the two."

Investigate thoroughly before participating in any non-traditional methods. Many of these so-called "miracle cures" can actually cause harm. For example, laetrile, touted as a cancer cure, has been shown to have no positive effect on cancer and can be, in fact, poisonous. Since its first use in the United States almost 40 years ago, there has not been a single scientifically documented case of it curing cancer.

In many cases, faddists' remedies are untested and merely exploit the vulnerable position in which patients and families find themselves when serious illness strikes. However, other therapies that fall outside the mantle of traditional medicine may have value in reducing pain, easing anxiety, or reducing side effects of traditional therapy. Recent studies on the positive effect of imagery, support groups and even hypnosis which focus on the body's ability to heal itself demonstrate that there is much we need to learn about non-medical approaches to healing.

The experimental therapies discussed above, such as vaccines and other types of immunotherapy, are very different from non-traditional or unproven methods. From preliminary animal studies to human clinical trials, experimental therapies are closely monitored by objective members of the medical community. Comprehensive data is collected and reviewed by critical observers to ensure safety and efficacy. On the other hand, unorthodox treatments such as laetrile, herbs, and other remedies do not undergo careful scrutiny.

Stories of a "miracle cure" may cause some desperate people to believe that the treatment is safe and effective. But unless large-scale studies have been done, one or two testimonies should not convince you that a non-traditional treatment works. Any patient considering alternative therapy should bear in mind the following:

- Alternative remedies are usually not tested on animals before being tried on humans.
- Occasional good results from alternative remedies often occur while the patient is undergoing traditional therapy.
- Alternative remedies are usually not reported in professional journals, which require careful analysis and peer review of the data before publication.

Before trying any alternative therapy, you should discuss your intentions with your doctors. He or she may be able to give you information about the risks involved. You may be able to work with your doctor and use alternative remedies while continuing conventional treatment. If you have to discontinue your conventional therapy to participate in an unorthodox one, this may be a compromise that is far too risky. You should be aware of the potential costs and uncertainty of faddists' remedies and scrutinize them carefully before trying any.

The American Cancer Society has a committee on unproven methods of cancer treatments that tracks the status of many claims of new treatments.

Worldwide Research Efforts

In March 1993, over 600 dermatologists, oncologists, surgeons, and biologists from around the world gathered in Venice, Italy, for the International Conference on Melanoma to discuss the latest breakthroughs in the causes, diagnosis, and treatment of the disease. From early morning until late afternoon, lectures and lively debates took place in cool damp auditoriums situated inside the Cypress Cloister on the small island of San Giorgio Maggiore, providing a serene and contemplative venue for the exchange of scientific ideas. Renaissance oil paintings hung in darkness inside the lecture halls as researchers presented their information with charts, graphs and photos, detailing the progress made in the three years since the last meeting.

Experts from around the world presented papers describing the outcomes of new therapies. The results of the studies were tiny steps forward in a journey of many miles. Detailed statistics sometimes obscured the fact that the real battle was being fought each day by individual patients who participated in the clinical trials being discussed. Many had braved the uncertain outcome and side effects of experimental treatments; others had not survived.

Despite the clinical atmosphere, a sense of urgency prevailed. It manifested itself in informal gatherings in hallways where intense discussions about new treatments lasted long after the lectures were through. Often a group of colleagues greeted one another warmly and then abruptly changed the subject to the business at hand. It was not a disease which held these attendees in such rapt concentration. Rather, it was the patients each doctor had seen and treated in a hospital or clinic and fervently wished to cure.

CHAPTER 13

Emotional Aspects of Melanoma

The biological aspects of melanoma are best understood by experts trained in specialized medical fields. The emotional part is uniquely understood by patients and those who love them.

While most patients are grateful to their doctors, especially the ones who are good at providing encouragement and support, a patient's emotional strength comes mainly from family, friends and, more importantly, him or herself.

Confronting Our Illness

Anatole Broyard, a writer who detailed his experience with prostate cancer, described his illness this way:

> *The knowledge that you are ill is one of the momentous experiences of your life. You expect that you are going to go on forever, that you're immortal. Freud said that every man is convinced of his own immortality. I certainly was. I had dawdled through life up to that point, and when the doctor told me I was ill it was like an immense electric shock. I felt galvanized. I was a new person. All of my old trivial selves fell away, and I was reduced to essence. I began to look around me with new eyes.*

There is little doubt that cancer can change a person. For some, like Nick Steiner, a diagnosis of cancer resulted in his looking at life in a different way and re-establishing priorities.

Nick Steiner, a family doctor with a specialty in cardiology, diagnosed and treated sick people for years, but admits he never completely appreciated how a patient with a serious disease felt until he learned he had melanoma. Twelve years ago, Nick had a successful and busy Park Avenue practice in New York. He was married with two children and seemed to have everything any person could want.

His wife noticed an unusual mole on the back side of his knee. Preoccupied with his patients and other responsibilities, Nick waited a few weeks before having the mole examined. He realizes in hindsight that his delay was more the result of denial than being too busy. Eventually, he saw a dermatologist who diagnosed the mole as malignant. Despite an excision of the 1.7 millimeter-thick nodular-type melanoma, the cancer reappeared. Nick believes denial during this time actually helped him cope with the rapidly unfolding events in his life. "Denial prevents you from letting your disease overwhelm you," he says.

As he recalls this turbulent period, Dr. Steiner is surprisingly calm, almost as if he were describing events that happened to someone else. In fact, Nick says that he is no longer the same person he was when he first found out about his melanoma. Faced with the idea that his very life was threatened by a disease that can be relentless, Nick reassessed everything. His lifestyle had become more of a burden than a pleasure. "The phone and the beeper were in charge and I was a slave to them," he now says.

The big problem was that he had not realized how unhappy his busy life had made him. Eventually his illness caused him to sell his practice. He characterizes himself as having been "cancer-prone, because I was so stressed out," during the time before he found out about his melanoma. In Nick's opinion, one of the reasons he developed melanoma was that his immune system was compromised by his unhappiness. He says one of the most stunning moments of revelation came to him when he was about to enter Memorial Sloan-Kettering Cancer Center for surgery because of a recurrence. "I felt relieved. I turned off my beeper, turned off the phone and I was practically whistling," he says. He realized that this inappropriate response to his situation meant that his disease was allowing him to give up the things he no longer wanted, and with that came an exhilarating liberation.

Now in his late 50s, Nick has fared much better than most melanoma patients with a recurrence, but the journey has been filled with many frightening downturns. In 1987, doctors discovered a brain tumor that was successfully removed, and in a separate operation a tumor in his stomach was removed. Nick has never received any chemotherapy or radiation.

He realizes that he has beat the odds. "I consider myself very fortunate to have done as well as I have," he says.

Many cancer patients describe their experience as a battle or a struggle, and for them, this turns out to be an effective method of fighting their disease. For Nick, melanoma has been an opportunity for self-awareness and the discovery of emotions he had bottled up inside himself for many years.

For the past few years, Nick has been participating in an experimental vaccine program offered by New York Medical College in Valhalla, New York. He is optimistic about the effect the vaccine is having on his body. He states that his blood tests indicate a very favorable response to the vaccine and he has no side effects from it.

Today, Nick is an avid photographer and also enjoys writing. The walls of his simple apartment are lined with his photos of natural landscapes and streaks of clouds. The hustle of New York, the beepers, the late night calls, the social whirl are memories. There is little regret in Nick's voice when he speaks about the life he had. He knows that he is fortunate, not just for having overcome a terrible disease, but for the positive effect it has had on his life. "In a sense, you could say that melanoma was the best thing that ever happened to me, in a weird way."

Twenty-two year old college student Matt echoes Nick's comments. Matt was diagnosed with melanoma that eventually spread to his lymph nodes, necessitating extensive surgery to his back and underarm. As a result of the surgery, he lost some movement in his back and was unable to fulfill his lifelong dream of becoming a sports physical therapist. Matt is now being treated with a tumor vaccine and chemotherapy. He views his experience with cancer as a challenge. His religious faith as well as his faith in himself has allowed him to put things in a positive light. "I think of it as a way to live that much better, to be a better person. If I live to be 95, I will appreciate every day."

Matt also believes family and friends are important. "If you have no support system, find one, because it comes in handy when you are fighting this disease."

An avid outdoor sports enthusiast, Matt says that he no longer goes out into the sun, but still finds ways to keep in shape. He has discovered two new hobbies—indoor swimming and spelunking. Finally, Matt is trying to stop asking himself "Why me?"—a common question with no answer for cancer patients. "I've got to do what I've got to do and the cancer is going to do what it's going to do," he said.

David, a 25-year-old graduate of the United States Air Force Academy, faced the recurrence of melanoma by using all available resources, including his own inner strength—strength that he never even realized he had before his illness. When David describes his experience with melanoma, his voice has the steady disciplined cadence of a military man. It belies the struggle that continues even today. In 1988, his sister-in-law noticed a mole on David's back and suggested that he have it checked. He saw a doctor who told him there was nothing to worry about. His mole itched and bled, but David thought nothing of it, especially because he wasn't able to see it. A year later, David was in the emergency room for a respiratory infection and a doctor there noticed the mole. David recalls that night. "I could tell right away that something was up because the first doctor who saw me started calling in all the other doctors." The emergency room doctor's suspicion was confirmed when the mole was removed and diagnosed as a 1.87 millimeter-thick melanoma.

David had never heard of melanoma. "I was surprised by the seriousness with which the docs were taking it. They told me I had to stay at the hospital. I did not have a clue about melanoma. I knew in general that moles could turn sour, but I wasn't aware there was a fatal type of skin cancer."

To David's relief, all the tests taken at the time showed no sign that the melanoma had spread anywhere else. David continued his service in the military, spending a year in California and then went to Korea. Although he said he felt well, he "never totally forgot about it."

On July 1, 1992, a doctor felt a small lump in David's left armpit. He was immediately scheduled for surgery. The doctors found ten malignant lymph nodes. He describes how he felt immediately after the surgery. "I woke up and had the feeling that things didn't go right. I looked up at the clock and saw it was five p.m., and I knew it should have been over a lot quicker. They told me what they found and the first thing I did was cry. I knew how serious it was and it set me back on my heels." Because of his condition, he was forced to go on medical retirement from the military, an idea that at first was unappealing to him because he loved being in the Air Force.

"Everything went downhill for about three months. I didn't have a job in the Air Force anymore, and I had too much time on my hands and wasted too much of it worrying."

David's initial fear and anger eventually subsided. "I thought, hey, I may only have a year left, and I'm not making much use of it. I started to think about it more and more, and I started getting used to the idea. I knew I would have to dedicate myself 100 percent of the time to beating this thing. I said if I don't start working on my will to live, it's going to kill me." He also realized that it was important to be with family and friends. He moved back to Ohio where his father, brother and sister-in-law live. Being with family members was helpful both emotionally and on a practical level. His brother escorted him to his chemotherapy treatments. "It made a difference just knowing he was with me," David says.

Eventually David found work as a drill instructor at a juvenile military camp for troubled youths, which he calls a "dream job." He is able to use his military experience to help teenagers with therapy and discipline. He says he loves helping children.

Besides finding the right emotional and psychological situation, David knew he needed the best medical care as well. He consulted with an Air Force physician, who told him there was nothing he could do because there was no proof that any treatment would really help him. David refused to accept that and set up an appointment on his own with a specialist in melanoma. The new doctor suggested a combination of chemotherapy and immunotherapy for David, who decided to try the treatment. "Although I knew some of the therapy would be harsh, I felt at least I am not going to be sitting on my butt waiting for this thing to re-appear."

In addition to his treatments, David has also adopted other lifestyle changes. He has re-entered a martial arts program, lifts weights every day, and has improved his diet. He also tries to maintain an upbeat perspective. "Even though it sounds difficult, try to keep your sense of humor. It is my strongest ally.

"I'm back in the living mode. First I read about the technical aspects, but now I read about the will to live. My number one goal is to be happy and to have as much fun with my life as possible. If I'm happy and having fun, I'm going to still be here, regardless of what the odds are. I've got a long way to go even though I've come so far."

Ginny, a Michigan social worker who was faced with a recurrence of her melanoma, says that it is important to keep a positive attitude, but not to close yourself off from the pain. She emphasizes the importance of allowing yourself adequate time to feel badly, to cry and to grieve. "You can't set your watch on your emotions," she says. "Remember to be patient and gentle with yourself. Allow the negative feelings to flow, so you can be free to experience all the positive things happening around you. They are there if you look for them."

Leaving Out Blame

Susan, a 30-year-old Wall Street executive, has been battling melanoma with considerable success since 1985. Susan remembers some therapists and even other cancer patients asking her why she wanted or needed her disease. Unlike other patients described in this book, Susan does not feel that her cancer changed her life in any positive way. "I needed this disease like I needed a hole in my head. I didn't feel like there was anything missing in my life before my diagnosis."

She also recalls being questioned by doctors about her prior sun exposure and being made to feel like she was partially to blame for having melanoma. Susan rejects these notions. "I can't change my having been in the sun, much of which happened when I was a child and didn't know any better." Susan's convictions have kept her focused on her goal—getting well.

She relied on certain psychological techniques to get her through difficult times in the course of her disease. "We did a lot of imaging. I'd lie down and listen to the tape, imagining there was a barrier forming around the cancer cells and squeezing them out. Someone drew pictures of PAC-Men coming for the cancer and placed them around my hospital room. I used them to form positive images of the treatment working."

She is cautious, however, about recommending these methods as a means to a cure. More importantly, she does not think that if a disease becomes worse a patient should feel responsible for not trying hard enough. Susan enjoyed imaging because it helped her to relax. She also had the emotional support of her husband, parents and friends. All of this contributed to keeping her spirits high during the rough and uncertain weeks at the hospital during treatment. Eventually, Susan's tumor responded to the therapy. "The fact that I got better wasn't simply because of my attitude. Saying that is too much like blaming people for their disease, and also blaming them if they don't get better. While it's important to keep a good outlook, it's not the only answer."

Although the mind has an a important impact on the body, it may be more productive to view healing and a good outcome as the result of a mixture of things—an optimistic patient, supportive family members, good doctors, effective medicine and some good luck. Blame should have no part in the process.

Physicians, too, need to do their part. Doctor Daniel Rosenblum writes in *A Time to Hear, A Time to Help*:

> *I believe we oncologists are responsible for listening well to all of our patients, whether they are optimists or pessimists. We ought not to judge the quality of the effort our patients are making to 'get well.' Rather it is our obligation to respond to their ailments and to discover the context within which they view their malignancies, their illnesses, and their lives.*

The Relationship Between the Mind and the Body in Melanoma

One author writing about cancer notes, "Without the admission of fear, courage is make-believe." One part of a six-year U.C.L.A. School of Medicine study of people with melanoma suggests that well-managed stress can sometimes play a positive role in the outcome of the disease. The authors of the study suggest that a realistic and healthy reaction to a diagnosis of cancer includes, at least initially, a degree of distress. This emotion, rather than being totally destructive, can often mobilize an individual—and may even play a role in increased survival.

The U.C.L.A. patients selected had either Stage I (no metastasis) or Stage II (local node metastasis) melanoma. After diagnosis, one group of patients participated in group meetings that consisted of education about melanoma and basic nutrition, stress management, enhancement of coping skills and psychological support. By the time this group had finished the program, they reported significantly less psychological distress and better coping strategies than those who had not been through the program.

What short-term tangible benefits did those who participated in stress management classes receive? Initially, they all reported less depression, fatigue, and confusion, as well as more energy—all positive changes that can make a great difference in day-to-day living. Six months after the support sessions, there was also evidence of increased levels of potential cancer-killing substances (Natural Killer Cells) in the bloodstream of patients participating in the stress reduction classes. Two-thirds of the patients participating in the classes had a 25 percent or more increase in cancer-fighting cells. There was no such increase in the control group.

The second part of the study, however, was the most dramatic, for it focused on actual survival. Of the 34 patients who had participated in the support groups, seven had recurrences and three had died. Of the 34 melanoma patients who did not participate in a support group, there were 13 recurrences and ten deaths.

These authors believe that minimizing our feelings about a cancer diagnosis may prevent the mobilization of coping resources and behaviors that are essential in dealing effectively with the physiological threat of a serious disease. They concluded that those patients who minimize the importance and threat of cancer appear to be at the greatest risk.

Before any definitive conclusions can be drawn about the positive effects of emotional support, long-range studies need to be conducted, but these early findings lend credence to the belief that the mind has a powerful influence on the body. The authors of the study believe that the large number of long-term survivors of melanoma who have features associated with a poor prognosis may owe their survival to such untraditional, interventional approaches.

Caring for a Loved One With Advanced Disease

Like other cancers, melanoma is a family illness. It often strikes people in their 30s and 40s, many of whom are parents of young children. What do these young ones need to know? Dr. Jon Levenson, a psychiatrist who specializes in the care of terminally ill patients, states that children need to know what is happening to adults they love. "Children personalize the illness and may believe that they did something wrong. They don't need to know all the details, but they should be told their parent is ill. By not discussing the situation, a child can begin to feel guilty and act out their anger and fear," he says.

Mike, an emergency room doctor in Van Nuys, California lost his wife Shelley to melanoma in 1992. She left behind two young children.

"The most important thing I can tell people is to involve the family. Don't separate yourself, don't make a wall," he says.

Shelley, a registered nurse, was diagnosed with metastatic melanoma in 1988 and underwent traditional, experimental and holistic therapy. When it appeared that her cancer was continuing to grow, her husband decided to take care of her at home so she could be with him, her children, and her parents and sisters.

The decision to keep a terminally ill person at home and out of the hospital is a difficult one. Mike was better equipped than most people to handle the physical details of his wife's care because of his training. Still, as he recalls the last few weeks of Shelley's life, he is moved to tears. No one is ever fully prepared for the emotional strain that this experience exacts. It requires a real effort on the part of the family to provide for the physical needs of the patient. More importantly, allowing someone to die at home takes a great deal of courage. For some, the effort is worthwhile.

Mike recalls that his children were involved in their mother's care during the last few months of her life and were present when she passed away. Shelley often spoke to the children in a way they could understand about what life would be like without her and she gave them advice about the future. Mike believes that his children have coped better with their mother's death because of their involvement with her illness.

For many reasons—financial, physical and emotional—a patient may prefer not to die at home. In other situations, a caretaker may need support from professionals experienced in caring for terminally ill patients. In either case, hospice programs can be helpful. In the United States, hospice programs can provide support for caregivers and dignity to patients either at home or at an in-patient facility. There are over 2,000 hospice programs in the United States. In 1992, they served 246,000 patients, 78 percent of whom had cancer. Caring for a terminally ill loved one is never easy, but the burden can be made lighter with the help of others.

Comforting Our Loved Ones

When melanoma does not respond to treatment and progresses, a patient and his or her family may need to come to terms with the possibility that cure is not possible. For some families, this idea is too difficult to accept, and everyone around the patient continues to say "I think you'll be fine," "This is just a minor setback," or "Don't worry." Lawrence LeShan, an expert on treating the emotional needs of cancer patients, writes: "What the dying person needs is someone to hear who they are and what their life has been. It is very easy to be reassuring—very easy and useless."

Physicians, as well, sometimes avoid discussing death with their patients because the subject is too difficult for them, especially if they need to shield themselves from the continual pain of suffering and death that they experience on a day-to-day basis. Dr. Levenson says: "Physicians are focused on cure and treatment. When there is nothing left to offer, they become uncomfortable discussing that. While it is devastating news to a patient that nothing is working, often a patient is most concerned about being abandoned. Patients understand that things are not going well. It is important to convey to them that while there is no further effective therapy, we will continue to work together to provide supportive care. I have often told oncologists that even though chemotherapy has stopped working, a patient may still need to see the doctor to address other issues like pain management and psychiatric needs."

Communicate your feelings to your doctor, especially if you feel you are not getting the emotional support you need. He or she may refer you to someone better equipped to deal with these problems. Dr. Levenson emphasizes that talking about your illness can reduce anxiety. "By expressing your worries, you may be able to get some distance from them. This should be part of the physician/patient relationship as well as the patient's relationship with loved ones," he says.

The Helping Hand

Human beings are social animals. They look to each other for comfort and companionship. When cancer strikes, people find great comfort in talking with other cancer patients. Cancer support groups cut back on feelings of isolation through a shared experience. Some support groups are highly organized, while others arise spontaneously when one person meets another who has similar experiences to share about an illness.

When Sharon Pratt was diagnosed with metastatic melanoma in 1986, she was unable to find understandable information about the disease or any guidance regarding experimental treatments. She wanted to reach out to other melanoma patients and connect with them, but soon found that there were no organized support groups for patients with melanoma. In 1988, she underwent treatment for the spread of her melanoma, and became even more frustrated over the lack of information about the disease. As she persisted in her struggle, she gradually met more and more people like herself who needed to talk about the anxieties and worries unique to melanoma.

In the spring of 1988, Sharon started "The Helping Hand," a newsletter that she single-handedly publishes from her home. "The Helping Hand" reaches out to over 5,000 melanoma patients in the United States and around the world. From this newsletter, a network of information and support has been created. Data on the latest experimental therapies, personal testimony from melanoma patients and helpful hints on sun protection make "The Helping Hand" a lifeline of emotional support.

Reaching Out

One melanoma patient who was interviewed for this book expressed gratitude at being able to tell her story. She said that just talking about her experience to someone else made her feel better. Everyone needs to start talking about melanoma. Those who are well need to tell others how to prevent and identify the disease. Those who have been stricken need to reach out and speak freely about their worries and concerns.

It is not easy to talk about a disease with someone who is

suffering—even if that person is close to us. However, people who are very ill need to have their condition acknowledged. If that means simply saying, "I'm sorry you are sick" or "How can I help?" that may be enough.

Until more effective and long-lasting treatment for advanced melanoma is discovered, the support of family and friends remains one of the most vital components of care. However difficult, it is an effort that benefits both patient and caregiver. The hardest part of communicating is most often listening. This is a challenge faced by everyone touched by this disease.

☼

CHAPTER 14

Safe Sun Habits for a Lifetime of Healthy Skin

Until the 1930s, a pale complexion was not only acceptable, but desirable in many cultures. Porcelain skin was a sign of aristocratic breeding, indicating the avoidance of outdoor labor. In centuries past, "sunburnt" meant rude and uncouth, since a red face was associated with work in the fields and peddling wares out of doors. Women of nobility covered their faces with paper or cloth masks before emerging outdoors, to avoid any color from the sun. Dark skin and ruddiness was dusted over with white face powders or blanched with lemon juice to achieve a pale countenance. Female American colonists, like many 17th and 18th Century women, used bonnets and parasols for protection against the sun's tanning rays.

Fashion designer Coco Chanel is attributed with popularizing a year-round tan in the first half of the 20th Century. Skin darkened by the sun became a status symbol as air travel permitted the wealthy to jet to resorts and bask on Mediterranean beaches. In the 1950s, air travel became less expensive and increasing numbers of tourists from cooler climates were able to vacation in sunny ones. Tans were in.

According to one author, "by the 1960s the superior femininity of lily-white skin had become an outdated concept, replaced by the healthful vision of the golden California girl..." These factors, as well as skimpier swim wear, exposed more and more people to risks associated with melanoma.

The "glow" of a suntan has became increasingly desirable over the years, to the dismay of modern dermatologists, who insist that there is no such thing as a "safe tan."

According to the American Academy of Dermatology, 25 percent of women they surveyed said they would not change their sun protection habits, even after learning about the relationship between melanoma and the sun. Americans spend an average of 1600 hours a year (about 30 hours a week) outside in the sunlight. Fortunately, bad sun habits are beginning to change. In the 1990s, the aesthetic cultural pendulum has swung back to pale, spurred in part by the pop icon Madonna. Her white skin has become a fashion statement.

No doubt both health and beauty considerations have played a role in people staying out of the sun. In a recent survey of 6,000 *Glamour* magazine readers, 89 percent reported that they now use sunscreen, and two-thirds of the respondents said they spend less time trying to get a tan now than they did five years ago. Fear of skin cancer was the reason cited by 69 percent and fear of wrinkles by 57 percent.

If you have fair skin, you have probably had a sunburn at some point in your life. This type of intense damage raises your risk for melanoma, especially if you were burned as a child or adolescent. Sunburns should be avoided completely. It is the intense intermittent damage that takes place during vacations, when your skin has been "undercover" for the greater part of the year that is linked to melanoma. If you tend to sunburn, your body is telling you that your skin and the sun don't mix. Take heed of the message. Keep in mind that the glow of a summer tan is a short-lived experience that will fade. The damage done to your skin, however, is permanent and irreversible. And the damage it does to your health could be life-threatening.

Ozone Depletion: One Part of
the Melanoma Time Bomb

The ozone layer is a naturally-occurring belt of gases in the stratosphere, ten to 30 miles above the Earth's surface. Intact, it absorbs almost 99 percent of ultraviolet B radiation before it reaches the earth. Scientists have chronicled the erosion of the ozone layer since the 1970s.

Some scientists fear that the depletion of the ozone layer will result in an increase of skin cancer, cataracts and impaired immune systems. Recent calculations estimate that every one percent decrease in the ozone layer is expected to increase the incidence of basal cell and squamous cell skin cancer by almost three percent. The Environmental Protection Agency predicts that there will be a 26 percent worldwide increase of skin cancer, including a five to eight percent increase in melanoma, by the year 2000 if depletion continues at current rates. For this reason, preserving the ozone layer is an essential part of skin cancer prevention.

Many studies have shown decreases in the ozone layer. Researchers report that the ozone layer was reduced by three percent in heavily populated areas of the northern hemisphere during 13 summers from 1979 to 1991, resulting in a six percent increase in UVB reaching the earth's surface. The change in ozone is due wholly or in part to the increased abundance of chlorofluorocarbons (CFCs), man-made chemicals that release chlorine and bromine into the atmosphere. In addition to CFCs, gas from volcanic eruptions also contributes to ozone depletion.

An international agreement known as the Montreal Protocol, signed by 23 nations in 1987, called for a 50 percent decrease in the use of CFCs by 1998 (compared with 1986 emissions). Subsequently, an amended Protocol to phase out all CFCs by the year 2000 was ratified by 64 nations. Large developing countries like China and India, however, have not stopped CFC production.

CFCs have been banned in the United States, Canada, Norway and Sweden for use in non-essential aerosols such as hairsprays and deodorants since 1978. They are still used in the United States and other countries, however, in many refrigerators, air conditioners, fire extinguishers and other products.

Individuals can do their part to save the ozone layer by not using polystyrene foam or any product packaged with it. Instead, use paper, glass or plastic. Insulation products that are manufactured in a way that harms the ozone layer (rigid urethane and isocyanurate) can be replaced with fiberglass, cellulose fiber and recycled wood fiber. Furthermore, you can purchase helium, water or alcohol-run refrigerators and air conditioners that run on evaporation and do not deplete the ozone layer (as opposed to traditional freon-run appliances). The Environmental Defense Fund, an organization that closely monitors ozone depletion, recommends that state and local governments establish centralized recycling centers to receive and reclaim refrigerants.

The depletion of the ozone layer makes it even more imperative for you to follow safe sun habits.

Personal Sun Protection

Noel Coward wrote of his countrymen, "Mad dogs and Englishmen stay out in the midday sun." The quote says a lot about the wisdom of retreating into the shade when the sun is at its strongest. Staying out of the sun, especially during midday, is by far the most effective way of reducing your risk of getting melanoma.

This advice, however, conflicts with most people's inherent love of the outdoors and activities like golfing, swimming and tennis. The fact is that almost everyone enjoys being outside in nice weather. The sun's warmth and brightness provide feelings of health and relaxation.

As one author has noted, however, sunlight can be "tonic or toxic" to human skin. As a tonic, the sun is responsible for photosynthesis, psoriasis treatment, and for warmth. Too much sun, on the other hand, causes skin cancer, wrinkles, cataracts, burns and sun allergies. Moderation, therefore, is essential so we can enjoy the sun's benefits but reduce its harmful effects.

Avoiding the midday sun (from 11 a.m. to 3 p.m. Daylight Savings Time or 10 a.m. to 2 p.m. Standard Time) is an intelligent compromise for those who simply cannot resist being outdoors.

Keep in mind that the amount of harmful radiation reaching your skin at any given time depends upon a variety of factors. The closer you are to the equator, the more potent the sun's rays. Increased altitude also increases UV radiation exposure; for every thousand feet above sea level you climb you are getting four to five percent more radiation. If you are a skier, keep your exposed skin protected with sunscreen. Just because it's cold outside doesn't mean the sun isn't reaching your skin. Snow reflects up to 80 percent of the sun's rays.

Clouds and haze can reduce the temperature, but not certain types of harmful UV radiation. Keep yourself covered, even on cloudy days.

Umbrellas are good sources of protection, but not as effective as hats and protective clothing. Umbrellas and parasols protect the skin from overhead light, but do not exclude ultraviolet light scattered from sand, water, snow and concrete. You may not be protected under an umbrella on the beach because of the reflective glare.

When planning a day outdoors, try to find a place where

there is a shady area available so you and your family can take cover during peak sun hours. Skin cancer prevention experts around the world are actively trying to encourage the planting of trees and construction of canopies in public spaces, especially playgrounds.

Sunbeds: The Newest Culprits

Sunbeds and tanning salons are the latest form of assault on healthy skin. Dr. Arthur Rhodes, of the University of Pittsburgh School of Medicine, calls them "an unregulated bad experiment." With over two million customers annually, the sunbed and tanning industry is growing. Studies show that the operators of these establishments are poorly trained, or not trained at all, and know little about their equipment and its associated risks.

In a survey of 20 tanning bed operators, 80 percent informed potential customers that they would not get skin cancer from artificial tanning. This advice is incorrect and provides a false sense of security to people who may not burn under the lights of a sunbed, but may be harming their skin nevertheless.

Studies show that tanning parlor operators are unaware that exposure to artificial light can cause severe skin reactions. Patrons on certain medications or diets who may be extra-sensitive to concentrated ultraviolet rays are rarely warned of this danger. In one case, a woman who drank a large amount of celery juice, which contains chemicals that cause light sensitivity, went to a tanning bed and suffered severe burns.

Many people use tanning salons to "get a base" or "prep their skin" before they go on vacation to a sunny climate. Most tanning salons use UVA light, which can increase pigment in people with naturally darker skin. Tanning from repeated exposures in a tanning salon provides only minimal protection against many other types of damage that the sun causes. In the long run, UVA light may actually contribute to wrinkles and brown spots. More importantly, UVA light works hand in hand with UVB light in causing skin cancer, according to Dr. Rhodes.

Because tanning parlors are a relatively new phenomenon, the data linking them with melanoma is preliminary, but associations between the two are already being made. From 1988 to 1990, researchers in Sweden studied 400 melanoma patients and 640 healthy people under the age of 30. They asked them about their exposure to sunbeds and sun lamps. The study concluded that melanoma patients had used sunbeds and sun lamps significantly more often than did healthy people. Several other studies also suggest that artificial tanning devices appear to increase the risk for melanoma.

Protective Clothing

Before the development of sunscreen, clothing was the only form of protection against the sun's damaging rays. Desert dwellers traditionally wore loose garments that covered their head, legs and arms to keep themselves cool and protected from the sun. Many continue this custom today. Photographs from the early 1900s show sunbathers modestly attired with socks, bonnets and long sleeves. Fashions and morals changed and less and less was covered up. It is not surprising that melanoma rates climbed as bathing suits shrank.

Protective clothing is advisable because unlike sunscreen, there is no need for reapplication or wondering whether the entire skin surface is covered. Just keep your shirt on and you *are* covered.

Two companies that specialize in sun-protective clothing are Sun Precautions and Frogwear. The president of Sun Precautions, Shaun Hughes, was diagnosed with melanoma in 1983. In order to enjoy outdoor activities while being protected, he developed a line of clothing which provides higher sun protection than many typical summer weight garments (see Appendix). Consumers should be wary of companies which claim their clothing filters out harmful radiation while allowing the sun's tanning rays to penetrate the fabric. Such claims are questionable, and even if they are true, you may be damaging your skin by wearing them in the sun without any additional protection.

The Skin Cancer Foundation offers these tips for safe sun clothing:

- Hold the fabric up to the sun or a light bulb. If the intensity of the visible light is decreased, the fabric will also decrease ultraviolet radiation.
- Keep in mind that dark colors like black, blue and purple are better at protecting your skin than lighter colors. Also wet shirts are more transparent and cling to the body, so they provide less protection. Keep a second dry T-shirt on hand if you plan to go into the water with your shirt on.
- Choose a hat that is made from closely woven material rather than a wicker or loose straw weave.
- Never work outdoors without a shirt. Wearing a loose shirt on a hot day will actually keep you cooler than going without a shirt.
- Wear a sunscreen beneath airy linen clothing, and remember to use sunscreen on any parts of your body that are not covered by clothing, especially if you plan to be outdoors all day.

Eye Protection

Sunlight can cause cataracts and retinal damage and is being investigated as a cause of ocular melanoma. Wearing sunglasses that absorb UVA and UVB rays is an essential part of your sun protection wardrobe. The Food and Drug Administration and the Sunglass Association of America have devised a labeling system to help you select the type of eye wear you need to protect your eyes. They have been categorized as follows:

Type of Eyeglass	Type of Protection
Cosmetic	Blocks at least 70% of UVB radiation and 20% of UVA. Recommended for "around town" or everyday use.
General Purpose	Blocks at least 95% of UVB and 60% of UVA. Recommended for use in any outdoor activities.
Special Purpose	Blocks at least 99% of UVB and 60% of UVA. Recommended for use in very bright environments.

Prescription sunglasses most commonly contain CR-39, a clear plastic that absorbs 100% of UVB rays. Other materials in prescription sunglasses absorb between 90 to 98% of UVA rays. With so much protection, sunglasses are not just a fashion statement, but an invaluable sun protection tool.

Sunscreens: An Application For Healthy Skin

Sunscreens are not a substitute for the safe sun habits described above. They are an additional safeguard and are not a license to spend long periods of time in the sun, especially if you are fair-skinned.

The most important thing to understand about sunscreens is that none of them are 100% effective. Moreover, a recent study suggests that sunscreens may not protect people from melanoma. Many experts believe that mere avoidance of sunburn through use of a sunscreen is inadequate to prevent melanoma. Other factors such as the sun's immunosuppressive effects may play a role in melanoma's development. Use them but don't get a false sense of security. Everyone, regardless of their skin type, will experience a sunburn if they stay out in the sun long enough.

History of Sunscreens

Various forms of sunscreen have been around since 1928, but it was not until 50 years later that the F.D.A. categorized sunscreens as drugs intended to protect the structure and function of the skin. During World War II, soldiers used a sunscreen known as "Red Vet Pet." It was made of iron oxide and petroleum jelly, a mixture that was thick, greasy and very unpleasant, but exceedingly effective. As the demand for sunscreens has grown, manufacturers have developed more elegant products that are easy to use and specially designed for all skin types. Sun protection products are big business. In 1990, Americans spent $524 million on them and projected sales for 1995 are $808 million.

New Developments

Concern over the confusing and sometimes misleading claims made by manufacturers has prompted the F.D.A. to completely re-examine the sunscreen industry. On May 12, 1993, the F.D.A. issued a tentative final monograph in which it proposed rules regulating the over-the-counter sale of sunscreens. After these guidelines are finalized, all sunscreen products will have to comply with standards of safety and effectiveness established by the F.D.A. and be labeled accordingly.

Some of the highlights of the study included the following

recommendations:

- Removing Padimate A from the approved list of sunscreen ingredients. This is because Padimate A has been found to cause irritations when skin is exposed to the sun.
- Eliminating use of the phrase "anti-aging" from sunscreen products since the F.D.A. considered those words to be misleading.
- Requiring all sunscreen products to bear labels about the sun's potential harm and the product's ability to protect users.
- Requiring sunscreen products to carry labeling and directions for water resistance.

What Sun Protection Factor (SPF) is Right for You?
To determine the degree of protection your sunscreen provides, use this formula: First, recall the shortest amount of time in the sun that caused you to develop a mild sunburn. Multiply this amount of time by the SPF of the sunscreen you wish to use. For example, it may take a fair-skinned person who is not using sunscreen only 15 minutes to get enough sun to cause a light sunburn. If this person were to use a sunscreen with an SPF of 10 it would take ten times longer (150 minutes) before he or she would develop the same mild sunburn. Remember that perspiration, water and friction can reduce the effectiveness of a sunscreen, so you should reapply it at least every two hours and more if you have been active.

Be aware that SPF protection claims on any sunscreen products are mainly the result of laboratory testing. Those conditions vary substantially from the real world, so you may need additional protection. There are a multitude of variables that can affect how long it takes for your skin to burn. For example, altitude, ambient temperature, recent exposure to the sun, pollution, wind, medications and the season can change the amount of time it takes for your skin to get a sunburn.

You should also know that SPF numbers relate only to the protection afforded against Ultraviolet B rays. Many experts believe that the SPF numbering system is misleading. They argue that SPF numbers relate only to protection from a sunburn, but are not related to preventing skin cancer. In Australia, sunscreen products are not labeled with SPF numbers.

Other concerns revolve around the question of how high an SPF a person really needs. Should people use an SPF of 40, 50 or 100? The F.D.A. thinks that the best compromise in this area is limiting the highest SPF to 30. Scientific evidence shows a point of diminishing returns for most people at levels above that number. According to the F.D.A., the difference in protection provided by a sunscreen with 40 or 50 SPF as compared with 30 "is so small as to be non-existent." Many experts disagree with the proposal to cap SPF at 30. They argue that protection above SPF 30 might be needed for some people with certain diseases or others on medications that make their skin sensitive to sun.

Partially in response to the criticism of the SPF system, the F.D.A. has proposed an alternative sun protection guide. Instead of using the amount of time you are out in the sun as a guide, they recommend that you use a strength of sunscreen according to your skin type.

The F.D.A. is recommending that the following guide appear in the labeling of all sunscreen products:

Sunburn and Tanning History	Recommended Sun Protection Product
Always burns easily; rarely tans	SPF 20 to 30
Always burns easily; tans minimally	SPF 12 to under 20
Burns moderately; tans gradually	SPF 8 to under 12
Burns minimally; always tans well	SPF 4 to under 8
Rarely burns; tans profusely	SPF 2 to under 4

Types of Sunscreens

There are two basic types of sunscreens—chemical and physical. *Chemical sunscreens* absorb ultraviolet radiation; *physical sunscreens* actually reflect and scatter it. Most chemical sunscreens contain ingredients that absorb ultraviolet B radiation. Newer types absorb some UVA and UVB rays.

A common sunscreen ingredient para-aminobenzoic acid (PABA) or its derivatives, called PABA esters, provides UVB radiation protection. One type of PABA ester, called Padimate A, has been dropped from the F.D.A.'s list of approved ingredients because it was found to cause irritations when the skin is exposed to sunlight.

Other common ingredients which protect against UVB radiation include cinnamates, salicylates and anthranilates. Be forewarned that if you are allergic to cinnamon, you may also have an allergic reaction to cinnamates.

Protection Against UVA Radiation

Benzophenones and other chemicals such as dibenzoyl methane absorb some types of UVA radiation. Initially, researchers thought that only ultraviolet B rays damaged the skin because UVB was responsible for producing a sunburn. As a result, sunscreens were rated only according to

Examples of Substances Used in Sunscreens

Group	Ingredient Example	Type	Protects Against
Esters of para aminobenzoic acid	Padimate-O	Chemical	UVB
Esters of cinnamic acid	Ethylhexyl p-methoxy cinnamate	Chemical	UVB+ some UVA
Benzophenones	Oxybenzone	Chemical	UVB+ some UVA
Titanium dioxide	Micronized titanium	Physical	UVB+ UVA
Salicylates	Homomenthyl salicylate	Chemical	UVB
Anthranilates	Menthyl anthranilate	Chemical	UVA

the protection they provided against UVB. Ultraviolet A rays were considered less harmful because they helped us develop a tan and didn't seem to burn our skin. New studies show that UVA radiation also damages the skin. UVA radiation penetrates the skin more deeply than UVB rays. Experts believe that it causes skin cancer and can suppress the immune system.

Faced with this mounting scientific evidence, the F.D.A. acknowledged that a way to label sunscreens describing UVA protection should be implemented. The American Academy of Dermatology also has commented that UVA protection claims for sunscreens should be standardized, meaning that the specific effect of UVA radiation that is blocked should be described. For complete protection, use a sunscreen product that blocks both UVA and UVB rays—

so-called "Broad Spectrum" sunscreens. Besides UVA and UVB protection ingredients, broad-spectrum sunscreens usually contain a physical blocker as well.

Physical sunscreens: The lifeguard on the beach with her nose coated with white goo is probably using a physical sunscreen. These products are sometimes referred to as "chemical-free" sunscreens, but this is really a misnomer because they do contain chemicals. Fair-skinned people and those who spend a lot of time in the sun should use physical sunscreens with a high SPF.

The most common ingredients in physical sunscreens are zinc oxide or titanium dioxide. These substances are excellent blockers of UVA and UVB radiation. Although physical blockers are fairly water resistant, they can "melt" in the sun and therefore need to be reapplied every two hours in the heat. In the past, people shied away from these products because they were sticky and unsightly. Now they have been reformulated so that they do not leave a white film on the skin after being applied.

Test Before You Buy
Before using a sunscreen, test it on a small patch of skin on the underside of your forearm. Some ingredients may irritate your skin. Continue to try others until you find one that you can wear comfortably. Lotions or creams are recommended for people with sensitive skin because clear formulations (gels) may contain alcohol which can be irritating.

On the other hand, gels are a good choice for teenagers or anyone with a tendency to develop acne because they are water-based. If you tend to break out, look for the word non-comedogenic, meaning the ingredients won't block your pores. Choose a sunscreen that suits your skin as well as your activity. There are waterproof and sweat-proof types for sports enthusiasts. Others are fragrance-free and hypoallergenic for people with allergies.

Types of Sunscreens for Different Activities

For Daily Use: SPF 6-15 in a facial moisturizer or make-up.

For Use on Beaches and Prolonged Sunbathing: Sweat and water-resistant with an SPF of 15 or greater.

For Recreational Use: Sweat- and water-resistant with an SPF between 15 and 30.

For Senior Citizens: Non-PABA, SPF 15-20

For Children: Moisturizing, Nonirritating, Non-PABA, Waterproof with an SPF of 15.

(Adapted from: Fitzpatrick, Thomas B. et al.,
Dermatology in General Medicine,
New York: McGraw Hill, 1993, p. 1706)

The ABCDs of Sun Protection

Just like the warning signs of melanoma have an easy to remember ABCD list, so do safe sun habits.

They are as follows:

Avoid unnecessary sun exposure to harmful ultraviolet radiation at mid-day.

Block sunlight by wearing protective clothing and broad-brimmed hats, and UV-opaque sunglasses.

Cover up with chemical or physical sunscreens when sun exposure is desirable or unavoidable.

Do not indulge in prolonged sunbathing or tanning salons.

Educate children as well as uninformed adults about good sun-protection habits and examine the skin regularly for moles and other changes.

(Adapted from Fitzpatrick, Dermatology in General Medicine, p. 1700)

Self-Tanning Creams, Bronzers and
Tanning Accelerators: How Safe?

For some people, no amount of information about sun damage will convince them that a tan isn't attractive. Fortunately, self-tanning products allow the die-hard tan lover to look tan without going into the sun. The main concern of dermatologists is that people who use self-tanning products realize that the appearance of a tan from a bronzing cream doesn't provide any protection against natural sunlight. Studies show that the majority of consumers expect sunburn protection from self-tanning products. The fact is, most of these products do not contain any sunscreen. Also keep in mind that even if self-tanning creams contain sunscreens, the protection is lost as soon as the cream is washed off even though you still look "tan."

Sunless tanning products contain a chemical called dihydroxyacetone (DHA), which is classified as a colorant. DHA, a type of sugar, gives the skin a brown color as the result of the skin's reaction to it and is considered to be safe. Newer self-tanning products which contain amino acids as well as DHA are also safe and effective. These newer formulations provide slower tans but the skin doesn't turn orangy, a common problem in earlier products.

Suntanning pills are not safe. They usually contain a chemical called canthaxanthin which enters the bloodstream after ingestion and is partially deposited in skin tissue. Although the F.D.A. has approved the use of this product in low levels as a color additive in food, it is not approved at any level to impart color to the human body. There have been reports of aplastic anemia, allergic reactions, stomach cramps, hepatitis, diarrhea and itching associated with these pills.

Finally, tan acceleration products can supposedly increase

a tanned look with the use of tyrosine, a naturally occurring enzyme that creates melanin. The F.D.A. has warned consumers that any product containing tyrosine claiming to accelerate the tanning process is an unapproved new drug and is not recommended.

Protecting Your Children

A child's skin is soft, smooth and beautiful. Why? One important reason is that it has not been exposed to years of sunlight. The American Academy of Dermatology, in conjunction with the American Cancer Society, has mounted a sun protection campaign aimed at children from kindergarten to third grade. Through the use of bright posters and activity sessions, teachers emphasize that children can have fun outdoors without hurting their skin.

Children need their parents' help when it comes to sun protection. Youngsters get 50 to 80 percent of their total lifetime sun exposure before their eighteenth birthday. It is during this period that adults should carefully monitor their children's sun exposure and teach safe sun habits. Blistering sunburns in childhood are a known risk factor for melanoma. In one study, people who took long vacations to sunny climates as children were found to be at an increased risk for melanoma as adults.

Childhood melanoma is rare, but sun protection should begin as early as possible because damage from the sun accumulates over a lifetime. Adults need to keep their children out of the sun as much as possible. Since doctors do not advise using sunscreen on children under six months, keep these little ones out of the sun altogether or cover their bodies when you go outdoors. There is nothing healthy about a tan child.

Educating your child about sun protection is important. Pediatric dermatologists recommend that you tell children if their shadow is shorter than they are to find some shade.

One of the most important things a parent can do is to set a good example. By observing your own safe sun habits, your child will learn the importance of covering up and using sunscreen outdoors.

Prevention Pays Off

You can lower your risk of melanoma at the same time you keep your skin looking young and healthy. In the coming years, doctors hope that campaigns aimed at educating the general public about melanoma will result in a decrease in its incidence and resulting deaths. Already the death rate from this disease is declining as the result of early detection in many parts of the world.

To continue this trend, every person, especially people at high risk because of skin type or family background, needs to know the best ways to avoid sun damage. A new generation of sunwise/melanoma-aware individuals will reap the benefits of this message. Hopefully, melanoma can become a "once fatal" disease like pneumonia and tuberculosis. This goal is possible if we look in the right places—our own skin—and stay out of dangerous ones—like tanning beds and the midday sun.

Glossary

Acquired nevi: A mole that a person is not born with, but develops later.

Actinic Keratosis: A rough, sometimes scaly, precancerous growth on the skin caused by long-term exposure to sunlight.

Adjuvant therapy: Treatment to prevent or delay a recurrence of cancer. It is given to patients after they have completed initial therapy (usually surgery or radiation) and who have no remaining evidence of disease.

Amelanotic melanoma: A rare type of melanoma which is white, pink or red, rather than black or brown in color.

Anemia: A deficiency of red blood cells which may cause weakness and pallor.

Aplastic anemia: A serious form of anemia which occurs when the bone marrow function is depressed.

Antibody: A protein produced by the immune system which circulates in the blood and helps to destroy foreign substances.

Antigen: A substance recognized as foreign and capable of inducing an immune response.

Asymmetry: Sides of differing shape.

Atypical nevus: An acquired mole that appears different from common moles. Atypical moles are generally larger than ordinary moles and may have irregular borders. An atypical nevus and a dysplastic nevus are the same thing.

Axilla, axillary: Underarm, the underarm area.

Basal cells: Cells found in the lowest part of the epidermis. These cells divide to produce new skin cells, replacing those that die and slough off the surface of the skin.

Basal cell carcinoma: Cancer of the basal cell.

Basal cell layer: The bottom layer of the epidermis.

Benign: Not cancerous. a benign growth is not malignant and does not spread to other parts of the body.

Bone marrow: The spongy material within the bones that produces red blood cells,white blood cells and platelets (the cells that help the blood clot).

Biopsy: Surgical removal of a small piece of tissue for microscopic examination.

Broad-spectrum sunscreen: Sunscreen that provides protection against UVB and UVA rays, usually containing chemical and physical blockers.

Cancer: A disease characterized by uncontrolled cell growth, often with, the ability of cells to spread to other parts of the body where they can destroy healthy tissue.

Carcinoma: A type of cancer.

Carcinogen: A cancer-causing agent.

Chemotherapy: Treatment with anti-cancer drugs.

Chlorofluorocarbons: Chemicals that destroy the ozone layer.

Clinical trial: Research conducted with patients, usually to evaluate a new treatment. Clinical trials usually take place after studies with animals are completed.

Congenital nevi: Moles that are present at birth. The presence of these moles may place a person at a higher-than-average risk for melanoma.

Curettage: Removal of tissue with a curette, which is an instrument with a curved sharp edge.

Cutaneous: Referring to the skin.

DNA: Deoxyribonucleic acid. The basic molecule of genetic material.

Dermatologist: A doctor specializing in the treatment of skin disorders.

Dermatopathologist: A doctor who specializes in diagnosing skin disease by looking at samples under the microscope.

Dermis: The second layer of the skin.

Dysplastic nevi: See atypical nevi

Epidemiology: The study of the incidence and spread of disease in a population and the factors that influence that disease.

Epidermis: The top (first) layer of the skin.

Gene: The smallest element of genetic material, made of DNA.

Host response: The reaction by the immune system to a disease, infection or substance recognized as foreign.

Immune system: The complex group of organs and cells that defend the body against infection and disease.

Immunotherapy: A new and experimental treatment for cancer which uses the body's own immune system to fight disease. Vaccines and other biological chemicals are used to stimulate the immune system to recognize and destroy cancer cells.

Incidence: The rate at which new cases of a disease occur in a population.

Inguinal: Pertaining to the groin.

In situ melanoma: Melanoma that is limited to the epidermis (top layer of the skin).

Interferon: A protein, usually produced by white blood cells, which has many effects on the immune system. It slows the rate of growth and division of cancer cells, causing them to become sluggish and die.

Interleukin-2: A substance produced by lymphocytes. It stimulates the growth of cells that are an important part of the body's immune system.

Intra-arterial regional infusion: Treatment in which anti-cancer drugs are put directly into an artery which supplies blood to a region of the body, usually an arm or leg.

Invasive melanoma: Melanoma that has penetrated from the epidermis into the dermis and thereby acquires a pathway for possible spread.

Isolated limb perfusion: Treatment in which blood is withdrawn from a patient, pumped through a machine which adds anti-cancer drugs, and returns it to the major artery supplying the limb being treated.

Lymphokine-Activated Killer cells (LAK cells): A lymphocyte that has been exposed to Interleukin-2 and develops the ability to kill cancer cells.

Lentigo: A flat, tan-to-brown colored patch on the skin, often caused by sun exposure.

Lesion: A change in a tissue or organ, often caused by disease. A skin lesion is a change on the skin that appears different from normal skin. A pigmented lesion is a change on the skin that has color different from surrounding skin.

Leukocyte: White blood cell.

Lymph: The almost colorless fluid that travels through the lymphatic system and carries cells that help fight infection and disease.

Lymphatic system: The tissue and organs that produce, carry and store cells that fight infection and disease. This system includes the bone marrow, spleen, thymus, lymph vessels and lymph nodes.

Lymphedema: A swelling of a body part caused by the abnormal accumulation of lymph fluid. It can often occur after surgical removal of lymph nodes.

Lymphocyte: A type of white blood cell that plays an important part in immune reactions.

Lymph nodes: Small bean-shaped organs located along the lymphatic system. Also called lymph glands.

Malignant: Cancerous, as opposed to benign.

Melanin: The pigment, or colored substance produced by melanocytes. Melanin gives the skin its color and helps protect it from the damaging effects of the sun.

Melanocyte: A special cell in the epidermis that produces pigment called melanin. Large clusters of melanocytes may appear on the skin as a mole.

Melanoma: Cancer that begins in a melanocyte. Melanoma often appears on the skin as a new or changing mole.

Metastasis: The spread of cancer cells from one part of the body to another.

Mole: A visible collection of melanocytes on the skin, also called a nevus.

Monoclonal antibody: A laboratory-produced antibody that can target a specific antigen, such as one on a tumor cell.

Needle aspiration: The removal of tissue with a hollow needle or tube.

Nevus: The medical term for clusters of melanocytes. A nevus on the skin is commonly called a mole.

Oncologist: A doctor who specializes in treating cancer.

Ozone layer: Part of the Earth's atmosphere in which there is a concentration of ozone, a form of oxygen which absorbs a large part of the sun's ultraviolet radiation.

Palpable: Perceptible by touch or feel.

Papillary dermis: Top portion of the dermis.

Pathologist: A doctor who specializes in diagnosing disease by examining tissues and cells under a microscope.

Photoaging: Wrinkles, lines, spots and other signs of aging that occur as the result of exposure to the sun.

Photodamage: Injury to the skin caused by exposure to ultraviolet radiation.

Phototypes: Categories of skin sensitivity to sunlight.

Platelet: A cell found within the blood important for clotting.

Precursor: A sign or symptom that heralds another.

Primary melanoma: The original melanoma.

Prognosis: The expected or probable outcome of a disease.

Radiation therapy: Treatment with high-energy x-rays to kill cancer cells.

Recombinant: Refers to the splicing together of pieces of DNA.

Recurrence: The return of cancer after its apparent disappearance or removal.

Red blood cells: The cells which carry oxygen in our bloodstream.

Regression: The partial or complete disappearance of a tumor. Spontaneous regression refers to the disappearance of a tumor without medical intervention.

Reticular dermis: Deeper portion of the dermis.

Risk factor: A substance or condition that is associated with an increased chance of getting a particular type of illness.

Side effect: An unintentional and undesirable effect of a drug or treatment.

Skin graft: Skin that is surgically moved from one part of the body to another.

Stratum corneum: Top layer of the epidermis comprised of dead skin cells, the layer of skin visible to the eye.

Squamous cell carcinoma: Cancer of the squamous cells.

Squamous cells: A type of cell found in the epidermis.

Staging: The process of determining the extent of a disease.

Clinical Staging: A description of cancer which includes the size of the tumor and the extent of spread, if any, to lymph nodes or other parts of the body from the original site.

Microstaging: A measurement of the thickness of a primary melanoma in millimeters and the determination of which level of skin the melanoma has reached.

Tumor-Infiltrating lymphocytes (TILs): Special cancer-fighting cells of the immune system that are found in tumors.

Ultraviolet radiation (UV radiation): Energy that comes in the form of rays from the sun. There are three types of UV radiation: UVA, UVB and UVC.

Vaccine: A preparation of an immune-stimulating antigen, often derived from a disease-causing substance (i.e. a portion of a cancer cell or virus) which stimulates the immune system to fight that disease or to prevent subsequent disease.

Virus: A tiny infectious particle, usually consisting of a piece of genetic code (i.e. DNA) and a protective coating, that can reproduce only by invading host cells.

Appendix

The following organizations can help you with information, support and medical care.

INFORMATION AND EDUCATION

American Academy of Dermatology
930 N. Meachum Road
P.O. Box 4014
Schaumburg, IL 60168-4014
(708) 330-0230

Professional society for dermatologists; provides information on sun protection for children in conjunction with the American Cancer Society; sponsors, with local hospitals, free skin cancer screening day each spring.

American Cancer Society
1599 Clifton Road N.E.
Atlanta, GA 30329
(800) ACS-2345
(404) 320-3333 (in Atlanta)

Supports research, conducts educational programs and offers many services to patients and families. To obtain information about services and activities in local areas call the 1-800 number.

The Cancer Information Service Office
(800)-4-CANCER
Hawaii: 524-1234, Washington, D.C. 806-5700

Provides up-to-date information about the latest clinical trials in cancer treatment, including melanoma. Utilizes Physician Data Query (PDQ), a computer database that gives quick and easy access to treatments and names of organizations and doctors involved in caring for people with cancer.

SUPPORT GROUPS

The Helping Hand
c/o Sharon Pratt
26 Belmont Street
Portland, ME 04101

A patient-run organization devoted to providing information and support to people with melanoma. Please do not phone. Send a letter requesting the newsletter. Contributions are appreciated.

Nevus Network
The Congenital Nevus Support Group
1400 S. Joyce Street
#C1201
Arlington, VA 22202
(703) 920-2349 or (405) 377-3403

Provides a network of support for those with congenital nevi and other rare nevus syndromes through letters, telephone calls and meetings. Generates a newsletter that shares medical and psychosocial information.

Well Spouse Foundation
P.O. Box 801
New York, NY 10023
(212) 724-7209

National network of support groups for caregivers of chronically ill spouses and partners.

Organic Whole Life Society (O.W.L.S.)
P.O. Box 403158
Hesperia, CA 92340
(619) 946-1611
   Organization co-founded by a melanoma patient that emphasizes nutrition, organic gardening and a healthy lifestyle for people with serious illness.

MEDICAL CONSUMER INFORMATION
The National Council Against Health Fraud, Inc.
P.O. Box 1276
Loma Linda, CA 92354
(909) 824-4690
   A non-profit organization comprised of health professionals, educators, researchers, attorneys and concerned citizens wishing to actively oppose misinformation, fraud and quackery in the health marketplace.

The Center for Medical Consumers
237 Thompson Street
New York, NY 10012-1090
(212) 674-7105
   Assists in helping patients makes informed choices about medical and health care. Provides information and resources people may need to understand medical conditions and get the best treatment. Publishes a newsletter called "Healthfacts" with latest findings from medical journals.

American Board of Medical Specialties
(800) 776-2378
   Provides information about board certification of physicians in 24 specialties, including dermatology, dermatopathology and oncology. This organization will not refer or recommend physicians, but will tell you if a particular physician that you are considering is board certified.

COUNSELING AND NURSING ASSISTANCE
Cancer Care, Inc.
National Cancer Foundation
1180 Avenue of the Americas
New York, NY 10036
(212) 221-3300

Provides some financial assistance for patients who need nursing care at home. Also provides professional counseling and planning for patients and families.

Visiting Nurses Association
107 East 70th Street
New York, NY 10021
(212) 794-9200
A non-profit organization that provides at-home nursing care in the New York area.

Chemo Care
1-800-55-CHEMO (Outside of Northern New Jersey)
(908) 233-1103 (Within Northern New Jersey)
(908) 233-7510 (Hearing Impaired)
One-to-one organization for people undergoing chemotherapy. Provides a network of patients who have had similar treatment.

CANCER PATIENT ADVOCACY GROUP
CAN ACT-Cancer Patient Action Alliance
26 College Place
Brooklyn, NY 11201
Beverly Zakarian, Director
(Please write for information)
An advocacy organization for cancer patients. CAN ACT is involved with accelerated F.D.A. approval for cancer therapy, assistance with reimbursement from insurance companies and other issues that affect the lives of cancer patients.

SPECIAL SERVICES
Lymphedema Services, P.C.
600 Alexander Road
Princeton, NJ 08453
(800) 882-9498
and
360 East 57th Street
New York, NY 10022
(800) 848-1015

Privately-run clinic that treats patients with lymphedema problems using Complete Decongestive Physiotherapy which includes, manual lymph drainage, bandaging and compression and other techniques. Treatment periods vary from one to 28 days.

National Lymphedema Network
2215 Post Street
San Francisco, CA 94115
(800) 541-3259
Provides information and treatment for people suffering from lymphedema.

TRANSPORTATION

Air Care Alliance
2132 Walnut Avenue
Venice, CA 90291
(800) 296-1217
An air transportation clearinghouse for cancer patients in need of treatment at distant locations. They work with the Corporate Angels Network (914) 328-1313 which provides free space on private aircraft when flights are available.

Wings of Freedom
2535 Lewisville-Clemmons Road
Clemmons, NC 27012
(919) 969-9122
Provides air transportation for cancer patients and families. Works with commercial airlines for reduced fares to transport family members to attend funerals of loved ones.

HOSPICE CARE

National Hospice Organization
1901 North Moore Street #901
Arlington, VA 22209
(800) 658-8898
A non-profit and trade organization that provides information on hospice services, both in-patient and at home.

MEDICAL CENTERS OFFERING MELANOMA VACCINES
Please note that each program has various and changing criteria for patients who will be accepted into a study.

Dr. Alan Houghton
Chief, Clinical Immunology
  Service
Memorial Sloan-Kettering
Cancer Center
1275 York Avenue
New York, NY 10021
Contact: Linda Williams,
Research Nurse Co-ordinator
c/o Dr. Alan Houghton
(212) 639-2233

Dr. Jean-Claude Bystryn
Professor, Department of
Dermatology
New York University Medical
Center
550 First Avenue
New York, NY 10016
(212) 889-3846

Dr. Abraham Mittelman
Director of Clinical Investigation
Division of Neoplastic Diseases
Department of Medicine
New York Medical College
Valhalla, NY 10595
(914) 285-8374

Dr. Donald L. Morton
John Wayne Cancer Institute
Saint John's Hospital and Health
  Care Center
1328 22nd Street
Santa Monica, CA 90404
(310) 449-5213

Dr. Hilliard Seigler
Duke University Medical Center
P.O. Box 3966
Durham, NC 27710
(919) 684-3942
Note: Must call within six weeks
of diagnosis or surgery.

PROTECTIVE CLOTHING
Frogskin, Inc.
Sun Protective Clothing, Inc.
P.O. Box 2030
Cameron Park, CA 95682
(800) 845-9531

Sun Precautions, Inc.
Clothing and Accessories for Sun Sensitive People
168 Denny Way
Seattle, WA 98109
(800) 882-7860

CANCER CENTERS IN THE UNITED STATES

A Comprehensive Cancer Center is a designation given by the National Cancer Institute to institutions which have fufilled the requirements that the center have a strong core of basic laboratory research in several scientific fields such as biology and molecular genetics, a strong program of clinical research, and an ability to transfer research findings into clinical practice.

Clinical Cancer Centers focus on both basic research and clinical research within the same institutional framework and frequently incorporate nearby affiliated clinical research institutions into their overall reseach programs.

Both types of institutions provide patient care and conduct research in the laboratory.

COMPREHENSIVE CANCER CENTERS

ALABAMA
University of Alabama
   at Birmingham
Comprehensive Cancer Center
Birmingham, Alabama
(205) 934-5077

ARIZONA
Arizona Cancer Center
University of Arizona
Tucson, Arizona
(602) 626-6372

CALIFORNIA
Kenneth Norris, Jr. Comprehensive
   Cancer Center
University of Southern California
Los Angeles, California
(213) 224-6600

Jonsson Comprehensive Cancer
   Center
University of California at
   Los Angeles
Los Angeles, California
(310) 825-5268
(800) 825-2631

USE/Norris Comprehensive Cancer
   Center
University of Southern California
Los Angeles, CA
(213) 226-2370

CONNECTICUT
Yale University Comprehensive
   Cancer Center
New Haven, Connecticutt
(203) 785-4095

DISTRICT OF COLUMBIA
Lombardi Cancer Research Center
Georgetown University Medical
   Center
Washington, D.C.
(202) 687-2110

FLORIDA
Sylvester Comprehensive Cancer
   Center
University of Miami Medical School
Miami, Florida
(305) 545-1000

MARYLAND
Johns Hopkins Oncology Center
Baltimore, Maryland
(410) 955-8964

MASSACHUSETTS
Dana-Farber Cancer Institute
Boston, Massachusetts
(617) 632-3476

MICHIGAN
Meyer L. Prentis Comprehensive
   Cancer Center of Metropolitan
   Detroit

Detroit, Michigan
(313) 745-4329

MINNESOTA
Mayo Comprehensive Cancer Center
Rochester, Minnesota
(507) 284-3413

NEW HAMPSHIRE
Norris Cotton Cancer Center
Dartmouth-Hitchcock
Medical Center
Hanover, New Hampshire
(603) 646-5505

NEW YORK
Memorial Sloan-Kettering
   Cancer Center
New York, New York
(800) 525-2225

Roswell Park Cancer Institute
Buffalo, New York
(800) 767-9355

Kaplan Comprehensive Cancer
   Center
New York University Medical
   Center
New York, New York
(212) 263-6485

NORTH CAROLINA
Duke Comprehensive Cancer Center
Durham, North Carolina
(919) 684-2748

Lineberger Cancer Research Center
University of North Carolina
Chapel Hill, North Carolina
(919) 966-4431

Comprehensive Cancer Center
Wake Forest University
Bowman Gray School of Medicine
Winston-Salem, North Carolina
(919) 748-4354

OHIO
Comprehensive Cancer Center
Ohio State University
Arthur G. James Cancer Hospital
Columbus, Ohio
(614) 293-4878
(800) 638-6996

PENNSYLVANIA
Fox Chase Cancer Center
Philadelphia, Pennsylvania
(215) 728-2570

University of Pennsylvania
   Cancer Center
Philadelphia, Pennsylvania
(215) 662-6364

Pittsburgh Cancer Institute
University of Pittsburgh
Pittsburgh, Pennsylvania
(800) 537-4063

TEXAS
M.D. Anderson Cancer Center
University of Texas
Houston, Texas
(713) 792-3245

VERMONT
Vermont Cancer Center
University of Vermont
Burlington, Vermont
(802) 656-4580

WASHINGTON
Fred Hutchison Cancer Research
   Center
Seattle, Washington
(206) 667-5000
(bone marrow transplant is primary
treatment offered)

WISCONSIN
Comprehensive Cancer Center
University of Wisconsin
Madison Wisconsin
(608) 263-8090

CLINICAL CANCER CENTERS

UCSD Cancer Center
University of California at San Diego
  Medical Center
(619) 543-6178

Beckman Research Institute
  City of Hope
Duarte, California
(818) 359-8111, ext. 2292

University of Colorado
  Cancer Center
University of Colorado
Health Sciences Center
Denver, Colorado
(303) 270-3007

University of Chicago Cancer
Research Center
Chicago, Illinois
(312) 702-9200

Lurie Cancer Center
Northwestern University
Chicago, IL
(312) 908-8400

Columbia Presbyterian Cancer
  Center
New York, NY
(212) 305-6905

Cancer Research Center
Albert Einstein College of Medicine
New York, NY
(212) 920-4826

University of Rochester
  Cancer Center
Rochester, New York
(716) 275-4911

Nelson Institute for Enivronmental
  Medicine
New York University
  Medical Center
New York, New York
(212) 340-5280

Ireland Cancer Research Center
Case Western Reserve University
Cleveland, Ohio
(216) 844-5432

St. Jude Children's
  Research Hospital
Memphis, Tennessee
(901) 522-0306

Institute for Cancer Research
  and Care
San Antonio, Texas
(512) 616-5798

Utah Regional Cancer Center
University of Utah Health Sciences
Center
Salt Lake City, Utah
(801) 581-4048

Massey Cancer Center
Medical College of Virginia
Richmond, Virginia
(804) 371-5116

The following list of doctors appeared in October 1992 *Good House-keeping* Magazine as the best melanoma doctors in the United States. The list was compiled by interviews with department chairpersons at major hospitals. To avoid bias, those who voted were asked not to name anyone at their own institution:

SURGEONS

Charles M. Balch, M.D.
M.D. Anderson Cancer Center
Houston, TX

Kirby I. Bland, M.D.
University of Florida
College of Medicine
Gainesville, FL

Blake Cady, M.D.
New England Deaconess
Hospital
Boston MA

Tapas K. DasGupta, M.D.
Humana Hospital/Michael Reese
Chicago, IL

Frederick R. Eilber, M.D.
UCLA School of Medicine
Los Angeles, CA

Constantine Karakousis, M.D.
Roswell Park Cancer Institute
Buffalo, NY

Alfred S. Ketcham, M.D.
University of Miami
School of Medicine
Miami, FL

Edward T. Krementz, M.D.
Tulane University School
of Medicine
New Orleans, LA

Donald L. Morton, M.D.
John Wayne Cancer Institute
Saint John's Hospital and Health
Center
Santa Monica, CA

Douglas S. Reintgen, M.D.
University of South Florida
College of Medicine
Tampa, FL

Steven A. Rosenberg, M.D.
National Cancer Institute
Bethesda, MD

Hilliard F. Seigler, M.D.
Duke University
Medical Center
Durham, NC

Carl M. Sutherland, M.D.
Tulane University
School of Medicine
New Orleans, LA

Marshall M. Urist, M.D.
University of Alabama
at Birmingham
Birmingham, AL

Harold J. Wanebo, M.D.
Brown University
Roger Williams Medical Center
Providence, RI

Dupont Guerry, M.D.
Hospital of the University of
  Pennsylvania
Philadelphia, PA

Alan N. Houghton, M.D.
Memorial Sloan-Kettering
  Cancer Center
New York, NY

John M. Kirkwood, M.D.
University of Pittsburgh
  Medical Center
Pittsburgh, PA

Michael J. Mastrangelo, M.D.
Thomas Jefferson University
  Hospital
Philadelphia, PA

Frank L. Meysken, Jr., M.D.
University of California, Irvine
  Clinical Cancer Center
Orange, CA

Malcolm Mitchell, M.D.
University of Southern California
  Comprehensive Cancer Center
Los Angeles, CA

Larry Nathanson, M.D.
Winthrop University Hospital
Mineola, NY

Selected References

Chapter One

Khlat, M., et al. "Mortality from melanoma in migrants to Australia:Variation by age at arrival and duration of stay," in *American Journal of Epidemiology*, 135:1103, 1992, p. 1103.

Koh, Edward. "Cutaneous Melanoma," in *The New England Journal of Medicine*, July 18, 1991, pp. 171-181.

Glass, Andrew, G., et al. "The Emerging Epidemic of Melanoma and Squamous Cell Skin Cancer," in *The Journal of the American Medical Association*, October 20, 1989, pp. 2097-2100.

Albert, Viccki, A., et al. "Years of potential life lost: Another indicator of the impact of cutaneous malignant melanoma on society," in *Journal of the American Academy of Dermatology*, Vol. 23, No. 2, August 1990, pp. 308-310.

Rigel, Darrell, S., et al., "The rate of malignant melanoma in the United States: Are we making an impact,?" in *Journal of the American Academy of Dermatology*, December, Vol. 17, No. 6, 1987, pp. 1050-1053.

"Expert Studies Malignant Melanoma Factors," Interview of Dr. Rona MacKie by Lawrence Schachner in *Dermatology Times*, Feb. 1993, p. 57

DeLeo, Vincent, *Photo-sensitivity* New York:Igaku-Shoin, 1992.

Urteaga, B. et al, "On the Antiquity of Melanoma," in *Cancer*, Vol. 19, May 1966, pp. 607-610.

Fitzpatrick, Thomas B. personal correspondence, March 21, 1993.

Holland, James, Editor *Cancer Medicine, Third Edition*, Philadelphia:Lea and Febiger, 1993.

Fitzpatrick, Thomas B. Editor, "Childhood Sun Exposure: The Melanoma Time Bomb," in *Dermatologic Capsule and Comment*, Nov/Dec. 1992. p. 1.

Fitzpatrick, Thomas B. ,et. al. *Color Atlas and Synopsis of Clinical Dermatology*, Second Edition, New York: McGraw-Hill, 1992.

Fitzpatrick, Thomas.B. ,et al. *Dermatology in General Medicine*, Fourth Edition, New York:McGraw-Hill, 1993.

Friedman, Robert, J.,et al. "Malignant Melanoma in the 1990s," in *CA-Cancer Journal for Physicians*, July/Aug. 1991, Vol. 41, p. 201.

"Dysplastic nevi and malignant melanoma: A patient's guide," The Skin Cancer Foundation, New York, NY, 1992.

"Cancer Facts & Figures-1993," American Cancer Society, Atlanta, GA.

Balch, Charles, et. al. *Cutaneous Melanoma* Philadelphia: J.B. Lippincott, 1992.

Chapter 2

Ehrlich, P. and Feldman, S. *The Race Bomb:Skin Color, Prejudice and Intelligence* New York:Quardrangle, 1977.

Updike, John. *Self-Consciousness* New York:Ballantine Books,1989.

Balch, Charles, et. al. *Cutaneous Melanoma* Philadelphia:J.B. Lippincott, 1992.

Montagu, Ashley. *Touching: The Human Significance of Skin* New York: Harper and Row, 1978.

Montagna, William, and Parakkal, Paul. *The Structure and Function of Skin Third Edition* New York: Academic Press, 1974.

Williams, William Carlos, compiled by Robert Coles *The Doctor Stories* New York: New Directions, 1984.

Sagarin, Edward, Editor. *Cosmetics, Science and Technology*, New York: Interscience,1957.

Rook, Arthur, et al. *Textbook of Dermatology, Fourth Edition*, Oxford: Blackwell Scientific Publications, 1988.

Chapter 3

Patterson, James, T. *The Dread Disease: Cancer and Modern American Culture* Cambridge: Harvard University Press, 1987.

Wilson, Jean, D., Editor, et al. *Harrison's Principles of Internal Medicine, Twelfth Edition*. New York: McGraw Hill, 1991.

McAllister, Robert, M., et al. *Cancer* New York: Basic Books, 1993.

DeVita, Vincent, T., Editor, et al. *Cancer:Principles and Practice of Oncology, Fourth Edition*, Philadelphia:J.B. Lippincott, 1993.

Robbins, Stanley, editor, et al. *Pathologic Basis of Disease* Philadelphia: W. B.Saunders, 1984.

Roach, Mary. "Sun Struck," in *Hippocrates Magazine*, May/June 1992, p. 33.

Pack, George, T. *Treatment of Cancer and Allied Diseases* New York: P.B. Hoebner, 1940.

Hemingway, Ernest. *The Old Man and The Sea*, New York: Macmillian, 1952.

Vardi, B., et al. "Orthodox Jews Have a Lower Incidence of Malignant Melanoma. A Note on the Potentially Protective Role of Traditional Clothing," in *Cancer*, Vol. 53, 1993, pp. 771-773 .

Wolf, P., et al. "Effect of Sunscreens and a DNA excision repair enzyme on ultraviolet radiation-induced inflammation, immune suppression, and cyclobutane pyrimidine dimer formation in mice, in *Journal of Investigative Dermatology*, 101:1993 pp. 523-527.

Diagram of Development of Melanoma: adapted from Leong, Stanley *Melanoma: Advances in Treatment*, Austin: R.G. Landes Company, 1992.

Chapter 4

Fitzpatrick, Thomas B., et al. *Dermatology in General Medicine Fourth Edition* New York: McGraw-Hill, 1993.

Friedman, Robert, J.,et al. "Malignant Melanoma in the 1990s," in *CA-Cancer Journal for Physicians*, July/Aug. 1991, Vol. 41, p. 201.

Chapter 5.

Campbell, Maude, L. "AAD Education and Screening Program Reaches Millions," in *Dermatology Times (Supplement)*, April 1993, p. S6.

Jancin, Bruce. "High-Profile Melanoma Screening Programs Paying Off in Australia," in *Skin and Allergy News*, Nov. 1993, p. 16.

Kenet, Robert, O. "Clinical Diagnosis of Pigmented Lesions Using Digital Epiluminescence Microscopy: Grading Protocol and Atlas," in *Archives of Dermatology*, February, 1993, pp. 157-174.

Koh, Howard, et al."Who discovers melanoma?" in *Journal of the American Academy of Dermatology*, June 1992, pp.

914-919.

Brownmiller, Susan. *Femininity* New York: Fawcett Columbine, 1983.

Chapter 6

Roenigk, Randall, K. and Roenigk, Henry, H. *Dermatologic Surgery* New York: Marcel Dekker, 1989.

DeVita, Vincent, T., Editor, et al. *Cancer:Principles and Practice of Oncology, Fourth Edition*, Philadelphia: J.B. Lippincott, 1993.

Pariser, Robert, J. "Skin biopsy:Lesion selection and optimal technique," in *Modern Medicine*, July, 1989, pp.82-90.

N.I.H. Consensus Conference, "Diagnosis and Treatment of Early Melanoma," in *Journal of the American Medical Association*, September 9, 1992, pp. 1314-1319.

Chapter 7

Parker, David. *Biographical Dictionary of American Sports Football*, New York: Greenwich Press, 1967.

"Diagnosis and Treatment of Early Melanoma," in *Journal of the American Medical Association*, September 9, 1992, Vol. 266, p. 1314.

Schultz, Stephen and Mastrangelo, Michael. "The Pathophysiology and Staging of Cutaneous Malignant Melanoma," in *Seminars in Oncology*, February 1989, pp. 27-33.

Ghussen F., et al. "The Value of Current Staging Systems for Melanoma of the Extremities," in *Cancer*, July 15, 1990, pp. 396-401.

Slinghuff, C., et al. "The Annual Risk of Melanoma Progression," in *Cancer*, 70:1992, pp. 1917-1927.

Beahrs, Oliver, H. *Manual for Staging of Cancer, Fourth Edition* Philadelphia: J.B. Lippincott, 1992.

Breslow 5-year survival chart, Adapted from: Balch, Charles, M. et. al., *Cutaneous Melanoma Second Edition* Philadelphia: J.B. Lippincott, 1992, p. 194

Rowley, Matthew and Cockerell, Clay. "Reliability of Prognostic Models in Malignant Melanoma," in *The American Journal of Dermatopathology*, Vol. 13, No. 5, 1991, pp. 431-437.

Ho, Vincent, C., et al. "Therapy for Cuta-

neous Melanoma," in *Journal of the American Academy of Dermatology*, Vol. 22, No. 2, February 1990, pp. 159-171.
Nathanson, Larry, Editor. *Current Research and Clinical Management of Melanoma* Boston: Kluwer Academic Publishers, 1993.
Melanoma Research, Abstracts from the Third International Conference on Melanoma, "Volume of malignant melanoma and neoangiogenesis," March 1993, p. 25.

Chapter 8
Balch, Charles, et. al. *Cutaneous Melanoma* Philadelphia:J.B. Lippincott, 1992.
DeVita, Vincent, T., editor, et al. *Cancer:Principles and Practice of Oncology, Fourth Edition*, Philadelphia:J.B. Lippincott 1993.
Morton, Donald, L., et al. "Improved Long-term Survival After Lymphadenectomy of Melanoma Metastatic to Regional Nodes," in *Annals of Surgery*, October 1991, pp. 491-501.
Morton, Donald, L. et al. "Management of Early-Stage Melanoma by Intraoperative Lymphatic Mapping and Selective Lymphadenectomy," in *Surgical Oncology Clinics of North America*, Vol. 1, Number 2, October 1992.
"Complete Decongestive Physiotherapy An Innovative and Logical Approach to Lymphedema," Lymphedema Services, P.C., 1991.
Drepper, H., et al. "Benefit of elective lymph node dissection in subgroups of melanoma patients," in *Cancer* 1993, pp. 741-748.

Chapter 9
Morra, Marion and Potts, Eve. *Choices: Realistic Alternatives in Cancer Treatment*, Avon Books: New York, NY, 1980.
Broyard, Anatole. *Intoxicated by my Illness*, New York:Clarkson, Potter Publishers, 1992.

Chapter 10
Balch, Charles, et. al. *Cutaneous Melanoma* Philadelphia:J.B. Lippincott, 1992.

DeVita, Vincent, T., Editor, et al. *Cancer:Principles and Practice of Oncology, Fourth Edition*, Philadelphia: J.B. Lippincott, 1993.
Heenan, P.J., et al. "The Effects of Surgical Treatment on Survival and Local Recurrence of Cutaneous Malignant Melanoma," in *Cancer*, January 15, 1992, pp. 441-426.
Ho, Vincent, C., et al. "Therapy for Cutaneous Melanoma," in *Journal of the American Academy of Dermatology*, Vol. 22, No. 2, February 1990, pp. 159-171.
N.I.H. Consensus Conference, "Diagnosis and Treatment of Early Melanoma," in *Journal of the American Medical Association*, September 9, 1992, pp. 1314-1319.
"Taking Time, Support for People With Cancer And The People Who Care About Them," N.I.H. Publication No. 92-2059, January 1992. p. 65.

Chapter 11
Perry, Michael, C., Editor. *The Chemotherapy Sourcebook* Baltimore :Williams and Wilkins, 1992.
DeVita, Vincent, T., Editor, et al. *Cancer:Principles and Practice of Oncology, Fourth Edition* Philadelphia: J.B. Lippincott, 1993.
Paget, Stephen. "The Distribution of Secondary Growths in Cancer of the Breast," in *The Lancet*, 1, 1889, pp. 571-573
Hart, Ian, R. " 'Seed and soil' revisited: mechanisms of site-specific metastasis," in *Cancer Metastasis Reviews*, Vol. 1, 1982.
Kennedy, B.J. "Evolution of Chemotherapy," in *CA-Cancer Journal for Clinicians*, September/October, 1991, pp. 261-263.
Melanoma Research Report, NIH Publication No. 92-3030, Feb. 1992.
Balch, Charles, et. al. *Cutaneous Melanoma* Philadelphia: J.B. Lippincott, 1992.
"Chemotherapy and You," NIH Publication No. 92-1136, December 1991.
Bruning, Nancy. *Coping with Chemotherapy*, New York: Ballantine Books, 1993.
McKay, Judith and Hirano, Nancee. *The Chemotherapy Survival Guide* Oakland: New Harbinger, 1993.
Grunberg, Steven, M. and Hesketh, Paul, J. "Control of Chemotherapy-Induced Emesis," in *The New England Journal of*

Medicine, December 9, 1993, pp. 1790-1795.

Chapter 12

DeVita, Vincent, T., editor, et al. *Cancer:Principles and Practice of Oncology, Fourth Edition,* J.B. Lippincott: Philadelphia, 1993.

Bottger, David, et. al. "Complete Spontaneous Regression of Cutaneous Primary Malignant Melanoma," in *Plastic and Reconstructive Surgery,* March 1992, pp. 548-553.

Avril, M.F., et al. "Regression of Primary Melanoma With Metastases," in *Cancer,* March 15, 1992, pp. 1377-1381.

Ceballos, Patricia, I. and Barnhill, Raymond, L. "Spontaneous Regression of Cutaneous Tumors," in *Advances in Dermatology,* St. Louis: Mosby, 1993.

Rosenberg, Steven A. *The Transformed Cell* New York: G.P. Putman's Sons, 1992.

Cartei, Giuseppe, et al. "Reduced lymphocyte subpopulations in patients with advanced or disseminated melanoma," in *Journal of the American Academy of Dermatology,* Vol. 28, 1993, pp. 738-743.

Morton, Donald, et al. "Active Specific Immunotherapy in Malignant Melanoma," in *Seminars in Surgical Oncology,* May 1989, pp. 420-425.

Bishop, Jerry E. "Scientist Races to Find Vaccine for Melanoma," in *The Wall Street Journal,* October 27, 1992, p.1.

Holland, James F. *Cancer Medicine,Third Edition* Philadelphia: Lea and Febiger, 1993.

Zagorsky, Ellen S. "Caring for Families Who Follow Alternative Health Care Practices," in *Pediatric Nursing,* January/February 1993, pp. 71-75.

Cassileth, Barrie, R. "Questionable Cancer Medicine," published by the American Cancer Society, Inc., reprinted from *Cancer Investigation,* 4:591-598, 1986.

Nealon, Eleanor, "What are Clinical Trials All About? NIH Publication No 92-2706, Reprinted June 1992.

Spingarn, Natalie Davis. *Hanging in There* New York: Stein and Day, 1982.

Chapter 13

Broyard, Anatole. *Intoxicated by My Illness* New York: Clarkson Potter Publishers, 1992.

Richards, Victor. *The Wayward Cell: Cancer* Berkeley:University of California Press, 1978.

Buckman, Robert. *I Don't Know What to Say How to Help and Support Someone Who is Dying* New York: Vintage Books, 1988.

LeShan, Lawrence. *Cancer as a Turning Point,* New York: Plume, 1990.

Mandell, Harvey and Spiro, Howard, editors. *When Doctors Get Sick,* New York: Plenum, 1987.

Spingarn, Natalie. *Hanging in There* New York: Stein and Day, 1982.

Rosenblum, Daniel. *A Time to Hear, A Time to Help* New York:The Free Press, 1993.

Fawzy, Fawzy I. "A Structured Psychiatric Intervention for Cancer Patients," in *Archives of General Psychiatry,* August 1990, pp.720-725.

Fawzy, Fawzy I. "Malignant Melanoma: Effects of an Early Structured Psychiatric Intervention, Coping, and Affective State on Recurrence and Survival Six Years Later," in *Archives of General Psychiatry,* September 1993, pp. 681-689.

Chapter 14

Brownmiller, Susan. *Femininity* New York:Fawcett Columbine, 1984.

Marks, Ronald. *Sun-damaged Skin* London:Martin Dunitz Ltd, 1992.

Heller, Tom, Editor. *Preventing Cancers,* Buckingham:Open University Press, 1992, "Malignant Melanoma-The Story Unfolds" by Rona M. MacKie

Fedor, Melissa, Editor. "Good-bye Summer Tan," in *Glamour,* May 1993.

"Protecting the Ozone Layer:What You Can Do," printed by the Environmental Defense Fund, 1988.

Roan, Sharon, L. *Ozone Crisis* New York: John Wiley & Sons, 1990.

Fitzpatrick, Thomas.B., et al. *Dermatology in General Medicine,Fourth Edition* New York: McGraw-Hill, 1993.

Kennedy, Sandra, H. "Tanning Salon Regulation and Inspection Poor," in *Dermatology Times,* January 1993, p.22.

Dial, William, F. "Self-tanning Products Found Safe;Yet Do Not Offer Sufficient Sun Protection," in *Cosmetic Dermatology for the Patient*, Vol. 1, No. 1, 1993.

Detjen, Jim. "Ozone Layer has eroded to record levels" in *The Philadelphia Inquirer*, April 23, 1993, p. 1.

Steven, William K. "Rise in Ultraviolet Rays Seen in North America," in *The New York Times*, Nov. 16, 1993.

Leary, Warren E. "Ozone-Harming Agents Reach a Record," in *The New York Times*, Feb. 4, 1992.

Fitzpatrick, Thomas, B. Editor. " 'Gearing Up' for the Effects of High-Intensity Solar UVB," in *Dermatologic Capsule and Comment*, March 1992, p.1

Melanoma Research, Abstracts from the Third International Conference on Melanoma, "The use of sunbeds/sunlamps and malignant melanoma in southern Sweden, March 1993, p.65.

Fairchild, A., et al."Safety information provided to customers of New York City suntanning salons," in *American Journal of Preventive Medicine*, November 1992, p9. 381-383.

Sun and Skin News, "Getting Sundressed." Vol. 8, No. 3, 1991.

Nightingale, Swea. "FDA Supported Sunglass Association of America UV Labeling Policy," (Press Release, March 19, 1992).

Federal Register, 21 CFR Part 352, et al., May 12, 1993, "Sunscreen Drug Products for Over-the-Counter Human Use," Tentative Final Monograph, Proposed Rule

DeLeo, Vincent A. *Photo-Sensitivity* New York:Igaku-Shoin, 1992.

Thompson, Sandra, Ph.D. "Reduction of Solar Keratoses by Regular Sunscreen Use," in *The New England Journal of Medicine*, October 14, 1993, pp.1147-1151.

Sunscreen Products-Evaluation and classification, published jointly by Standards Australia, Standards New Zealand, 1993.

Fitzpatrick, Thomas.B., et al. *Dermatology in General Medicine. Fourth Edition*, New York:McGraw-Hill, 1993.

Ackerman, A. Bernard. "No one should die of malignant melanoma," in *The Journal of the American Academy of Dermatology*, Vol. 12, 1985, pp. 115-116.

Note:

Many sections of *Saving Your Skin* describe the personal experiences of people faced with a diagnosis of melanoma. Almost every person we asked gave us permission to use his or her name in the book. In some cases, however, we have chosen to use only first names and/or to transpose events or alter identifying characteristics.

Index

A

ABCD's of Melanoma, 42-44
Acquired nevi, 12
Acral-lentiginous melanoma, 50
Actinic keratosis, 54
Adjuvant therapy, 66, 128
  candidates for, 129
  trials, 80
A.J.C.C./U.I.C.C. Staging System,
  75-76
Albino, Anthony, 28, 37
Alternative therapy, 142-144
Amelanotic melanoma, 51
American Academy of Dermatology,
  162, 174, 178
American Cancer Society, 81, 105,
  121, 123, 144, 178
Anaplasia, 29
Anemia, 22, 122
Anthranilates, 173
Anti-nausea drugs, 120
Antibodies, 133
Antigens, 135
Asymmetry, 44
Atypical nevi, 14
Axilla, 90
Axillary dissection, 95

B

Basal cell carcinoma, 52
Basal cell layer, 25
Basal cells, 25, 52
Bathing trunk nevi, 14
BCG (Bacillus Calmette-Guerin),
  134, 136
BCNU (chemotherapeutic drugs),
  116, 119
Benzophenones, 173
Biopsy, 63-64
  techniques not recommended, 64

Biopsy for melanoma, 63
Blood test, 105
Bloodless biopsy, 59
Blue nevus, 54
Board certified, 82
Bone pain, persistent, 106
Boron neutron capture therapy
  (BNCT), 142
Boston University School of
  Medicine, 58-59
Breslow, Alexander, 71
Breslow microstaging for melanoma,
  71-73
Brownmiller, Susan, 58-59
Broyard, Anatole, 85, 146
Bruning, Nancy, 118, 124, 127
Burkitt's lymphoma, 33
Bystryn, Jean-Claude, 134-137

C

Cancer, causes of, 30-35
Cancer cells, growth rate of, 109-110
Cancer support groups, 159-160
Cancer Treatment Centers
  (see appendix), 124
Cancer vaccine, 127
Cancers, common characteristics of,
  29-30
Canthaxanthin, 178
Carcinogenesis, 30
Carcinogens, 32
Carswell, Robert, 5
Cataracts, 164, 166, 170
CCNU, 119
Chemotherapy, 80, 100, 107,
  112-113
  adjuvant, 114
  for advanced melanoma, 114-117
  combination, 116-117
  Dartmouth Regime, 116-117
  Dacarbazine (DTIC), 114-115, 120,
  121, 139

dangers of, 112
Fotemustine, 115
and immunotherapy, 118
method of delivery, 123
single-agent, 114-116
Taxol, 115
therapeutic, 114
Chemotherapy nurses, 124-125
Chemotherapy side effects, 119-123
anemia, 122
bleeding, 122
blood clotting problems, 123
hair loss, 121
infection, 122
nausea and vomiting, 119-121
other, 121-123
Children
and exposure to sun, 7
protecting against sunburn, 178
Chloroflourocarbons (CFCs),
163-164
Cinnamates, 173
Cinnamon, and allergy to sunscreens
containing cinnamates, 173
Cisplatin, 116
Clark, Wallace Jr., 72
Clark's Levels, 72-73
Clinical staging, 73-74
tests to determine, 76
clinical staging and microstaging,
combining, 74-76
Clinical trials, 129-130
discontinuing participation in, 129
questions before entering, 129
specific local information for, 130
Clothing, safe sun, 169
Collagen, 25-26
Color variegation, 43
Columbia-Presbyterian Medical
Center, 103, 119
Compound nevus, 53
Comprehensive Cancer Treatment

Centers (see Appendix), 124
Congenital nevi, 14
Coping with Chemotherapy, 118
Corporate Angels Network, 137
Cosmetic removal, 57
Cutancous melanoma, 17
Curretage, 64
Cyclophosphamide (Cytoxan), 136
Cyrosurgery, 52
Cytotoxic drugs, 113, 114

D
Dacarbazine (DTIC), 114-115, 119-
120
sidc effects, 115
Dartmouth Regime, 116-117
Dermatologist, 58, 62, 79, 80
Dermatology in General Medicine, 11,
176
Dermatopathologist, 64, 80
Dermis, 24, 25
Development of Melanoma, 42
Diameter, 45
Dibenzoyl methane, 174
Dihydroxyacetone (DHA), 177
Distant metastasis, 73, 106
Distant recurrence, 106
DNA (deoxyribonucleic acid), 27,
30-31, 34, 138
Doctor
affiliation of, 82
experience of, 82
and experimental therapy, 82
patient, family, 83-84
questions for, 82-83
Doctors, changing, 84-87
Drug evaluation, phases of, 130-131
DTIC (see Chemotherapy)
Dying
at home, 158
hospice care, 158
Dysplastic nevus, 13

E

Early detection, as secondary prevention, 1

Education, importance of in early detection, 17

Elastin, 26

Elective lymph node dissection (ELND), 91-94, 97

patient types for, 93

ELM

digital, 57

(see Epiluminescence microscopy)

Enlargement, 45

Environmental and lifestyle factors, 35-36

Environmental Defense Fund, 164

Environmental Protection Agency, 163

Epidemiology, 33, 36

Epidermis, 24, 27, 41, 98

Epiluminescence microscopy, 56-57

Ethnic background, 11-12

Ethnic groups at risk

Asians, 49

Blacks, 27, 49, 53

Caucasians 4,6, 8, 11, 26-27

Hispanics, 52

Native Americans, 52

Excisional biopsy, 63

Experimental therapies

faddist or questionable remedies, 142-146

future of, 141-142

interferon, 138-139

interferon-alpha 2B, 139

interleukin-2, 139-141

monclonal antibodies, 141

monitoring of, 144

Experimental therapy, 82, 101, 106

choosing, 128-129

Eye protection, 169

F

Fair skin, 27, 163

and exposure to sun, 7

and sunscreens, 176

Familial Atypical Mole and Melanoma (FAM-M) Syndrome, 13

Family history, 9, 18

Family history, how to prepare, 148

Fidler, Isaiah J., 108

Fitzpatrick, Thomas, 10-11, 16-17, 62

Five-year survival chart, 75

Food and Drug Administration (FDA), 115, 170, 171-173

Fotemustine, 116

Friedman, R.J., 78

Frogwear, 168

G

Gene, 32, 109

Genetic

makeup, 7

predisposition, 32, 41

George Washington University, 71

H

Hair loss, 121

Headache, 106, 110

Helping Hand, The (newsletter), 159

Hemingway, Ernest, 35

Hepatitis B virus, 33

Herbalism, 142

Hodgkin's disease, 114

Holism, 142

Homeopathy, 142

Hormonal agents, 112

Hospice

care, 84

programs, 157

Host response, 133

Houghton, Alan, 91, 99, 108, 115, 118, 129, 141

Hughes, Shaun, 168
Human skin, cross-section of, 28
Human skin phototypes, 11
Hypnosis, 143

I
Immune deficiency, 41
Immune stimulants, injections of, 99
Immune system, 25, 26, 89, 97, 127
  impaired, 164
  influence of on melanoma, 78
  spontaneous regression, 133-134
  workings of, 131-132
Immunologic drugs, 100, 112
Immunotherapy, 106, 128
  goal of, 132-133
  melanoma vaccines, 134
  non-specific immunostimulants, 134
  specific immunotherapy, 134-136
  types of, 134-136
In situ melanoma (see Melanoma in
  situ)
In-transit recurrent tumors, 100
Incisional biopsy, 63
Infections
  how to avoid, 122
  signs of, 122
Inguinal lymph node dissection, 94
Inguinal region, 90
Interferon, 133, 138-139
Interleukin-2, 134, 139-140
Intra-arterial regional infusion, 102
Investigational trial, 127
Ionizing radiation, 41
Isolated limb perfusion, 101-102

J
Jaundice, 22
John Wayne Cancer Institute, 94,
  136

K
Kenet, Robert, 57
Kinetic resistance, 113
Kirkwood, John M., 139

L
Laetrile, 143
Langerhans cells, 25
Lentigo, 56
Lentigo maligna, 14, 41, 50, 54
LeShan, Lawrence, 157
Lesion, 55, 98
Leukemia, 34, 112
Leukocyte, 139
Levenson, Jon, 103, 156, 158
Local disease, 73
Local recurrence, 98, 100
Lumps, in skin, 107
Lung cancer, 34
Lymph, 89
Lymph node dissection, 89-97, 101
Lymph vessels, 27, 89
Lymphatic mapping, 94-95
Lymphatic system, 89, 90
Lymphedema, 94-97
  and diet, 96-97
Lymphocytes, 132, 139
  B-lymphocytes, 132
  T-lymphocytes, 132
Lymphokine Activated Killer (LAK)
  cell, 139-140

M
Malignant cells, 108-109
Mastrangelo, Michael, 96, 117, 118
Mayo, Charles H., 28
Mayo Clinic, 28, 94
McGovern, Mary Patricia, 119
McKie, Rona, 10
M.D. Anderson Cancer Center, 108
Medical oncologist, 80, 81
Megestgrol acetate (Megase), 117

Melanin, 26, 37
Melanocytes, 26-27, 37, 39, 40
Melanoma, 14, 35, 114, 165
  among Blacks, Asians, Hispanics
  and Native Americans, 52
    appearance of, 51
  and chemotherapy, 117
  and children, 178-179
  as curable cancer, 3
  in Australia, 5-7
  causes, 36-37
  development of, 41
  early characteristics, 16
  emotional aspects of, 146-160
  evaluation, 74
  familial, 33
  as a family illness, 157-158
  fear of, 29
  highest incidence of, 6
  history of, 5
  how it spreads, 71, 106-108
  identification of, 44
  importance of removal, 65
  invasive, 41, 73
  in Israel, 38
  lifetime risk in United States t., 4
  and lymph system, 88-89
  ocular, 170
  protection against, 164-179
  preventing return of, 65-66
  recurrence of, 97-98
  return of, 2
  in Scotland, 38
  spread of, 107-111
  statistics on, 3-5
  steps to reduce deaths from, 17-18
  superficial spreading, 49
  survival of, 69
  thickness of, 69
  types of, 52-53
  and vitiligo, 141
Melanoma and the sun, 39-41, 161-
  162, 164-166
Melanoma from an unknown primary, 53
Melanoma in situ, 3, 40, 42, 92
Melanoma per 100,00 persons, 8
Melanoma Program and Melanoma
  Immunotherapy Clinic at New
    York University, 134
Melanoma recurrence, factors for, 97
Melanoma Risk Factors, 7-9
melanoma skin types, high risk, 11
Memorial Sloan-Kettering Cancer
  Center, 28, 91, 99, 108, 129, 141,
  148
Metastasis, 29, 40, 108, 110
Metastatic melanoma, traditional
treatment for
  chemotherapy, 112-113
  radiation, 111
  surgery, 111
Metoclopramide (Reglan), 120
Micrometastases, 115
Microstaging, 71-74
Mind and body, relationship of in
melanoma, 155-158
Moles
  atypical, 13-14, 40
  benign, 40, 57
  bleeding, 16
  changes in, 45-46
  hidden, 57
  importance in occurences, 40
  large or irregular, 40
  other high risk, 14-15
  small, 58
Moles and melanoma, 12
Monoclonal antibody, 140-141
Montagu, Ashley, 23
Montreal Protocol, 163
Morton, Donald, 94-95, 136
MRI, 77
Mucosal melanoma, 51

Mustard gas, 34, 111-112
Mutation, 110

N
Nathanson, Larry, 99, 107, 111, 117
National Cancer Institute, 81, 105,
  120, 124, 129, 130, 131
  Cancer Information Service, 131
National Cancer Intutite, Surgery
  Branch, 140
National Institutes of Health (NIH),
  13, 77, 86, 99, 142
Natural Killer Cells, 140, 155
needle aspiration, 90
Nerve dysfunction, 94
Nevus, 12
New York Medical College, 149
New York University, Melanoma
  Cooperative Group, 4
New York University School of
  Medicine, 78
Node dissection, side effects of, (see
  Lymph Node)
Nodular melanoma, 50
Norris, William, 5, 9
Nuclear scan, 76

O
Ocular melanoma, 51
Office of Alternative Medicine
  (O.A.M.), 142-143
Oncogenes, 30-31, 34, 110
Oncogenic transformation, 31
Oncologist, 98, 159
Oncology nurse, 119
Ondansetron (Zofran), 120
Oral contraceptives, 16
Ozone depletion, 164-165

P
PABA esters, 173
Padimate A, 171, 173

Paget, Stephen, 109
Papilliary dermis, 25
Para-aminobenzioc acid (PABA), 173
Pathologist, 64
  general, 79
Pediatric dermatologist, 180
Phillip, Arthur, 6
Photoaging, 10
Photographs, full body, 14
Photosynthesis, 166
Physical examination, 76, 105
Physical sunscreens, 173, 175
Pigmented lesion, 53
Plastic surgeon, 79
Pott, Sir Percival, 32
Pratt, Sharon, 159
Precautions, general, 95-96
Precursor lesion, 13, 49
Pregnancy and melanoma, 15-16
Prevention, need for, 180
Primary lesion, 64
Primary melanoma, 64, 74-75, 91,
  99-100, 110
  location of, 77
  thick, 80
Primary tumor, growth of, 107
Prochlorperazine (Compazine), 120
Prognosis, 22, 69-71, 74
  related to age, 77
  and sex, 77
Prognostic, factors for, 76
Prophylactic dissection, 89
Protective clothing, 13, 39, 167-168

R
Radiation, 81, 106, 111-112
Radiation oncologist, 81
Radiation therapy, 99
Recombinant DNA technology, 138
Recurrence, 98-101
Regional metastasis, 73
Regional recurrence, 101

Regression, 70, 133
Research efforts, worldwide, 145-146
Reticular dermis, 25, 27, 73
Rhodes, Arthur, 37-39, 59, 62,
  166-167
Risk factor, 8, 162, 168
Rosenberg, Steven A., 132, 140
Rosenblum, Daniel, 154

S
Salicylates, 173
Scar, 66
Seborrheic keratosis, 54
Second opinion, 64
Seed and soil theory, 109
Self examination, 14
Self-examination, 61
  importance of, 59-60
Self-tanning creams, bronzers and
  tanning accelerators,
  safety of, 177
Skin
  anatomy of
    dermis, 26-27
    epidermis, 25-26
  appearance of, 20
  human, structure and function of,
    25-28
  as organ, 19
Skin: key to our emotions, 23-24
Skin cancer, 166
  increase of, 164
  other types, 53-55
  prevention suggestions, 166-167
Skin Cancer Foundation, 13-14
  on safe sun clothing, 168
Skin graft, 66
Skin lesions, common, 53-54
Skin phototypes, 11
Skip metastasis, 94
Skolnick, Mark H., 32

Smoking, avoidance of in healing, 66
Southern Methodist University, 93
Spontaneous regression, 133
Squamous cell carcinoma, 52-53
Squamous cell skin cancer, 164
Staging, 70-72
Steiner, Nick, 146-149
Stratum corneum, 24, 27
Sun
  allergies, 166
  exposure, 10, 18, 27, 55, 104
  and melanoma, 39
Sun Precautions Inc., 168
Sun protection, as primary
  prevention, 1
Sun protection ABCDs, 177
Sun Protections Factor (SPF)
Sunbeds and tanning salons, 166-167
Sunblock, 39
Sunburn, 10, 163, 166
  avoidance of to prevent return of
    melanoma, 66
  and skin types, 10-11
Sunglass labeling system, 170
Sunless tanning products, 178-179
Sunlight, 35, 39, 53
  exposure, 51
Sun's radiation and it's effect on the
  human skin, 38
Sunscreen, 13, 166, 169-176
  broad-spectrum, 176
  chemical, 173
  chemical-free, 175
  examples of substances used in, 174
  F.D.A. guide for SPFs, 174
  history of, 170
  labeling, 171-172
  new developments, 170-171
  non-comedogenic, 175
Sun Protection Factor (SPF),
  172-173
  types for different activities,

170-171
 types of, 174-176
Suntanning pills, 178
Support groups, 156-157
Surgery, 106, 110-111, 127
Surgical oncologist, 65
Systemic chemotherapy, 99

T

Tamoxifen, 116, 117
Tanning, 27, 162
Tanning parlors (see also Sunbeds),
 168
Taxol (paclitaxel), 117
Therapeutic lymph node dissection,
 90-91
Thomas Jefferson University
 Hospital, 96
Titanium dioxide, 174
*Touching: The Human Significance of
 the Skin*, 23
The Transformed Cell, 132
Treatment, choosing, 118-126
Treatment of scars after melanoma
 excision, 66-67
Trials, to prevent a recurrence,
 129-146
Tumor-associated blood vessels, 77
Tumor infiltrating lymphocytes
 (TIL), 139
Tumor suppressor genes, 31, 110
Tumor thickness
 as relevant factor for prognosis, 72
 and survival, 71-72
Tumor volume, 77-78
Tyrosine, 179

U
U.C.L.A. School of Medicine, 154
Ulceration, 77
Ultraviolet A radiation (UVA), 35-36,
 166, 167, 173-175

Ultraviolet B radiation (UVB), 35-37,
 163, 167, 172, 173
Ultraviolet light, 27, 35, 54
Ultraviolet radiation, 7, 35-37, 39,
 41, 165
Union Internationale Contre le
 Cancer (U.I.C.C), 74
Univeristy of Utah Medical Center,
 32
University of Pennsylvania Medical
 School, 72
University of Pittsburgh School of
 Medicine, 37, 38, 59, 62
University of Texas, 9
Updike, John, 21
UV protective clothing, 166

V
Vaccine, 134-136
Vincristine, 121
Viruses, 33-34, 53, 136
Visiting Nurse Association, 123
Vitamins, 66
Vitiligo, and melanoma, 141

W
Weight loss, 106
Williams, William Carlos, 21-22
Winthrop University Hospital, 98
Wood's lamp, 77
World Health Organization
 Melanoma Group, 94

X
X-rays, 40, 52, 77, 106

Z
Zinc oxide, 176